D0515301

ABSOLUTE BEGINNER'S GUIDE

TO

Coaching Youth Soccer

Tom Hanlon

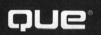

800 East 96th Street
Indianapolis, Indiana 46240

Absolute Beginner's Guide to Coaching Youth Soccer

International Standard Book Number: 0-7897-3359-5

Library of Congress Catalog Card Number: 2004118405

Printed in the United States of America

First Printing: June 2005

08   07   06   05   4   3   2   1

Trademarks

All terms mentioned in this book that are known to be trademarks or service marks have been appropriately capitalized. Que Publishing cannot attest to the accuracy of this information. Use of a term in this book should not be regarded as affecting the validity of any trademark or service mark.

Warning and Disclaimer

Every effort has been made to make this book as complete and as accurate as possible, but no warranty or fitness is implied. The information provided is on an "as is" basis. The author and the publisher shall have neither liability nor responsibility to any person or entity with respect to any loss or damages arising from the information contained in this book.

Bulk Sales

Que Publishing offers excellent discounts on this book when ordered in quantity for bulk purchases or special sales. For more information, please contact

U.S. Corporate and Government Sales
1-800-382-3419
corpsales@pearsontechgroup.com

For sales outside the United States, please contact

International Sales
international@pearsoned.com

Publisher
Paul Boger

Executive Editor
Candace Hall

Acquisitions Editor
Jeff Riley

Development Editors
Sean Dixon
Steve Rowe

Managing Editor
Charlotte Clapp

Project Editor
Tonya Simpson

Production Editor
Megan Wade

Proofreader
Andy Beaster

Technical Consultant
Peter O'Scanaill

Publishing Coordinator
Pamalee Nelson

Book Designer
Anne Jones

Page Layout
Susan Geiselman

Graphics
Laura Robbins

Photographer
Clark Brooks,
The Photo News

Contents at a Glance

Table of Contents

About the Author

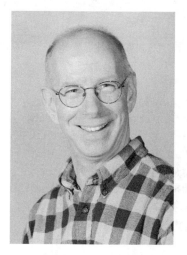

Tom Hanlon has 19 years of professional writing experience as a journalist, an editor of two coaching magazines, a curriculum writer for a coaching division of a publishing company, and a book writer and ghost writer for nationally prominent authors. Tom ghostwrote *Teens Can Make It Happen* (Simon & Schuster) for Stedman Graham; this book made the *New York Times* bestseller list in 2000. He has written all or major portions of 39 other books, including 7 sport officiating guides, numerous coaches' guides (for sports such as baseball, softball, soccer, basketball, and volleyball, among others), and a wide assortment of related sports titles. Tom is a full-time self-employed writer with considerable experience in writing books related to sports. He has played numerous sports himself and has experience as a youth sport coach.

About the Technical Consultant

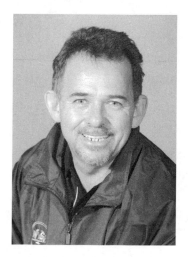

Peter O'Scanaill has played soccer at the high school and college levels as well as professionally for the Golden Eagles in Phoenix, Arizona. He played for, coached, and managed the Long Beach Tigers in California, and has been a player and manager of two over-30 men's teams. He is the travel commissioner for the Westfield Youth Soccer Association's boys travel program. He lives in Indianapolis.

Dedication

To all the youth soccer coaches who volunteer their time to teach kids the great game of soccer.

Acknowledgments

Many people used their talents to make this book happen. First and foremost, Jeff Riley, executive editor, paved the way for this book, inviting me to write it and getting it approved. Steve Rowe and Sean Dixon, developmental editors, provided consistently excellent advice in shaping the content and in making the book as useful and practical as possible. Tonya Simpson, project editor, managed all the details and tasks that go into developing a book and guided it through the process. Megan Wade lent her considerable talents as a copy editor, cleaning up and tightening the copy. And Peter O'Scanaill, the travel commissioner for Westfield (Indiana) Youth Soccer Association, provided his expertise throughout the project and created the games and drills in Chapter 11. A great thank you also to Clark Brooks of The Photo News for his expert camera work; his photos really helped show the skills in action.

We Want to Hear from You!

As the reader of this book, *you* are our most important critic and commentator. We value your opinion and want to know what we're doing right, what we could do better, what areas you'd like to see us publish in, and any other words of wisdom you're willing to pass our way.

As an executive editor for Que, I welcome your comments. You can email or write me directly to let me know what you did or didn't like about this book—as well as what we can do to make our books better.

Please note that I cannot help you with technical problems related to the topic of this book. We do have a User Services group, however, where I will forward specific technical questions related to the book.

When you write, please be sure to include this book's title and author as well as your name, email address, and phone number. I will carefully review your comments and share them with the author and editors who worked on the book.

Email: feedback@quepublishing.com

Mail: Candace Hall
        Executive Editor
        Que Publishing
        800 East 96th Street
        Indianapolis, IN 46240 USA

For more information about this book or another Que title, visit our website at www.quepublishing.com. Type the ISBN (excluding hyphens) or the title of a book in the Search field to find the page you're looking for.

Introduction

It all began so innocently.

Just as the youth soccer league administrator asked for a volunteer to coach your son's team, you scratched the top of your head. All the other parents were studying, with sudden keen interest, their thumbnails or shoelaces. No eyes, except yours, were looking forward.

The administrator saw her chance.

"Excellent! We have a new coach!"

To your astonishment, you saw that she was pointing directly at you. Parents, with relieved looks on their faces, turned to look at you. Some smirked. A few chuckled. All were joyful.

"Relax," one parent said. "The season doesn't start till next week."

"My kid's a striker. That's the only position he plays," another parent said as he gave you a good view of the bulldog tattooed on his bicep.

"My son plays sweeper," another parent added, as if he bought his son the position from Major League Soccer, which had granted the boy sole rights to play sweeper on your team.

"I never knew you could coach, Dad," your son said as you walked to your car.

"Sure I can coach," you said. "How difficult can it be?" You hoped you at least *sounded* convincing.

Every spring and fall, all across America, youth soccer leagues swing into action. Every year, thousands upon thousands of new coaches are tabbed to guide the players. The majority of those coaches have little or no experience coaching.

If you are one of those coaches, this book is for you. It is intended primarily for coaches of players from 6 to 12 years old, but it is applicable to coaches of older players as well. Use it as your rudder to guide you through your season. Use this book to

- Understand your role, and know what to expect, as a coach.
- Know the keys to being a good coach.
- Realize why kids play sports and consider how this should affect your approach to coaching.

- Bone up on the basic rules of soccer and learn how to impart those rules to your players.
- Provide for kids' safety and respond to emergency situations.
- Learn the general principles of teaching skills and tactics.
- Teach individual skills and team tactics.
- Coach effectively during games.
- Make the sport experience a meaningful and enjoyable one for the kids.
- Communicate effectively with parents, league administrators, referees, and players.
- Form positive alliances with parents, involving them in various ways.
- Plan for your season and your practices.
- Discover the keys to conducting productive practices.
- Celebrate victories and learn from defeats.
- Keep it all in perspective.

This guide presents the foundational concepts that effective coaches follow, and it shows you, step-by-step, how to incorporate those concepts, plan your season, and conduct your practices. It provides many forms you will need, including sample and blank season and practice plans, a sample letter to parents, an injury report and emergency information card, and a season evaluation form. It has games and drills you can use to teach your players the skills and tactics they need to know. It details how to execute the fundamental skills and tactics, so you will know what to teach—and it lays out *how* to teach. It is also replete with practical tips that will help your season be a success.

How This Book Is Organized

This book is organized in three parts. Part I, "Coaching Basics," provides guidance in a number of areas, including your basic approach to coaching, communication keys, safety principles, and practice planning. Part II, "Skills and Tactics," delves into the specifics of the skills and tactics your players will need to learn, ending with an entire chapter devoted to games and drills you can use to teach those skills and tactics.

Part III, "Appendixes," are six appendixes that you should find useful. This material includes a sample letter to parents, a medical emergency form, an injury report, blank season and practice plans you can use for your own planning, and a season evaluation form you can use at the end of your season.

Special Elements

Throughout the book you will find the following special elements:

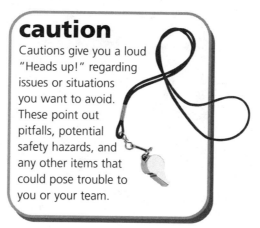

note

This is a note element. Notes give you relevant information that doesn't necessarily fit in the text flow.

tip

Tips are given to help you do something more efficiently or to give you the "inside" view on how to accomplish something related to coaching soccer.

caution

Cautions give you a loud "Heads up!" regarding issues or situations you want to avoid. These point out pitfalls, potential safety hazards, and any other items that could pose trouble to you or your team.

PART

i

COACHING BASICS

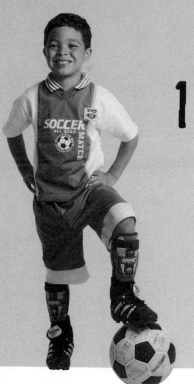

1

YOUR COACHING APPROACH

So you're a coach! Excellent. Most likely, you have a week or so to prepare for your first practice. But it's not time to jump into practice planning yet. Just as you will want your players to develop their fundamental skills first, you need to develop your basic coaching approach. Consider this chapter as your own personal coaching preparation. It provides the foundation for you to build upon.

Your Coaching Philosophy

When Charles Dickens began *A Tale of Two Cities* with "It was the best of times, it was the worst of times, it was the season of Light, it was the season of Darkness…", he wasn't describing the typical youth league season, but he could have been.

Competition can bring out the best in us, and it can bring out the worst in us. You've read the stories of coaches fighting with other coaches or with 16-year-old referees. You've probably witnessed parents screaming at the referees or at opposing players—or at their own kids. It doesn't happen all the time, but it happens often enough, even at the earliest levels of competition.

And it happens because of an overemphasis on winning. Our society places a premium on winning, and generally on winning at all costs. "Just win, baby," was the motto coined by Oakland Raiders owner Al Davis. This motto is fine at the professional level. It is *not* fine at the youth level. Why? Because when your focus is solely on winning, it comes at the expense of the kids you coach.

When your primary goal is to have an undefeated season or to win your league title, what happens? Every decision you make is based on whether it will help you win. So, you play Colin, Seth, and Max, your least-skilled players, as little as your league rules allow. You never play them in crucial situations, and you place Kendra only on defense, and instruct Zach, a much better defender, to do his best to cover for himself as well as for Kendra.

At the professional level, at the collegiate and high school levels, and even at upper youth levels, there's nothing wrong with this. At the lower youth levels, certainly at ages 6–12, plenty is wrong with it.

That overemphasis on winning comes at the cost of the kids' development and of their love for the game. It results in low morale when players don't win enough games to meet your, or their parents', expectations. It certainly discourages the lesser-skilled players, who thought they were going to play a game but find that their main duty is to stand on the sidelines and cheer on their teammates. It sends the message to kids that if they don't win, they have failed in their mission.

But their mission when they are 6–12 years old is to learn the game, to acquire and improve their skills, and to gain in their understanding of the rules and tactics. It is not to pummel the opponent, to make a name for themselves in the local media, or to win every title in sight.

Your approach, then, should be to develop the whole player in these ways: physically, mentally, emotionally, and socially.

tip

Remember, the only way kids are going to improve their skills is by receiving good instruction and playing the game. At this level, that's your mission: to give everyone solid instruction and playing experience.

Physical Development

It's your task as a coach to help your players acquire and develop the physical skills they need to perform. You need to teach them the basics: dribbling, passing, receiving, heading, shooting, marking, tackling, and goalkeeping.

In Chapter 6, "Player Development," you'll learn how to teach skills and tactics. Chapter 9, "Offensive Skills and Tactics," and Chapter 10, "Defensive Skills and Tactics," are devoted to the correct execution of the skills and tactics you will be teaching, so you'll know step-by-step how to demonstrate proper execution.

Players' physical development is one of the obvious duties of a coach, and one that takes preeminence in practice. But practices and games can be used to develop players in other ways as well, including their mental development.

Mental Development

Justin makes a great tackle and heads downfield with the ball. He spots Sam, a teammate, who is hanging back by the opposing goalkeeper, with only the goalie between him and the goal. Justin rifles a pass to Sam, who deftly receives the ball and kicks it in for the apparent score. He is overjoyed, but his joy is drained when the referee whistles and calls offside, negating the goal. You sigh and make a note to teach—or reteach—your players about the offside rule at your next practice.

Especially at the youth level, kids won't know all the rules and they won't know many—if any—of the strategies of the game. If you teach skills in the context of how your players will use them in a game and tell them why they need to know how to do the skill, chances are they will retain the *why* part. Also be aware that they might not understand these items the first few times you tell them, but as you continue to teach and remind them, it should sink in.

One of the greatest joys of coaching is seeing that your players know what to do in game situations. When your players begin to understand and execute the basic concepts of good spacing, of moving to open areas, of forming a triangle to support the player with the ball, and of moving continuously, you will be thrilled. And so will they because, in understanding and executing these concepts, they will significantly improve as a team.

This won't happen all at once, and some of it might not happen at all at the youngest levels. But if you clearly and simply explain the basic tactics and help them understand the game and how to respond to various situations, their mental development is fun to watch. The mark of a good team, especially at the youth level, is not that they execute every play perfectly, but that they know what they should be trying to do in each situation.

Emotional Development

Each player is a unique person. Some players are outgoing; some are reserved. Some are excitable; some are laid-back. Some are jokers; some are serious. Some have trouble listening or paying attention; others soak in most of what you say.

As a coach it is crucial that you understand that any one approach won't work the same with each child. Ann might be fine with some gentle kidding, whereas Alex might be bothered by the same kidding. Get to know your players as best you can in the first few weeks, and instruct and encourage them in the ways that will help them be ready and eager to learn and to play.

Remember that games produce situations that can become quite emotional for players (not to mention coaches!). Some players will be disconsolate after a loss; others won't be bothered at all. Help keep your players on an even keel. We talk more about how to do so in Chapter 7, "Game Time!"

Social Development

Soccer is great for social development. It takes a team effort to win. Players must rely on each other, pull for each other, and learn how to play with each other as they strive to win.

Use teachable moments to emphasize the team aspect of soccer. Such moments include an opportunity for a give-and-go play, setting up or defending a corner kick, spreading out the offense, coming over to help a defender, and so on. Each situation involves teammates and each is executed for the good of the team.

Reinforce team unity in practices and at games. Don't treat "star" players differently. Look to enfold "fringe" players, those who are quiet or less-skilled and who might otherwise go unnoticed, in all team aspects. Also, be sure to emphasize the importance of everyone's contributions and point out those contributions when they happen.

Some Final Thoughts on Your Coaching Philosophy

Winning is a worthy goal, and one you should pursue as a team. However, as a youth soccer coach, winning cannot be the ultimate goal. The physical, mental, emotional, and social development of each player should be your ultimate goal, and winning should be secondary.

When you develop your players' physical talents and mental abilities, you are putting them in a position to win. Teach them the game and its rules and tactics so they will be prepared to perform to the best of their abilities and knowledge. Encourage your players; let them know it's okay to make mistakes, and to learn from those mistakes.

When you focus on developing the whole player, that doesn't mean you're necessarily going to win your league or have a high winning percentage. It means you're keeping winning in its proper place—as a byproduct of sound player development, keeping each child's best interests at heart.

Sound difficult? It's not, if you develop the attributes of a good coach.

10 Attributes of a Good Coach

Just as your players are unique individuals, so are coaches. Maybe you're an extrovert; maybe you're an introvert. Maybe you're in a leadership position at work and are used to supervising people; maybe you have no supervisory experience at all. Regardless of your background, you can be an excellent youth soccer coach if you develop the following 10 attributes:

- Take your role seriously—but not *too* seriously.
- Be comfortable with being in charge.
- Be dependable and stable.
- Be patient.
- Be flexible.
- Enjoy getting to know your players.
- Desire to help kids learn and grow.
- Be an encourager.
- Be willing to learn.
- Have a sense of humor.

Let's take a brief look at each attribute.

Take Your Role Seriously

Now that you have volunteered to coach, commit yourself to the time and energy it will take to coach. Showing up on time at the practice field or for the game is not enough. Show up prepared to conduct the practice, prepared to coach your players during the game, and ready to instruct and supervise your players. Your role is to teach your players how to play soccer. They're looking to learn from you.

On the other hand, keep things in their proper perspective. These are games, learning experiences—and are intended to be *fun* learning experiences—for kids who are 6–12 years old. Their soccer experience generally *is* fun, win or lose, unless it is tarnished by overzealous coaches or parents who place such a great emphasis on winning that all the fun drains out of the game.

Keep the fun in the game. Keep the kids' best interests at heart. Relax; take a deep breath; enjoy the sunshine; and focus on the task at hand, such as how to pass the ball, how to shoot, or how to mark or tackle.

Use your players as a guide. If they look tense or are unusually quiet at practice, or if they're avoiding your look, they're probably taking their cues from you, and you'd better lighten up your approach. On the other hand, if they're cracking jokes and goofing off and aren't focusing on the task at hand, you need to gain control. You'll learn some tips on how to do so in Chapter 5, "Practice Plans."

Ultimately what you're after is a steady pace at practice where learning and fun are synonymous and ongoing.

Be Comfortable with Being in Charge

Every child will be looking to you for instruction. You have to be comfortable with being the leader, the teacher, and the resident expert who knows how to instruct and conduct effective practices. There's a fine line between having fun at practice and simply goofing off. You need to know what your goal is in each practice, and you need to steer your kids in that direction while maintaining an open and friendly atmosphere within that context.

If you're not comfortable being in charge and are unable to set the proper tone for practice, one of two things happens: Either the practice crumbles into chaos and nothing is learned as kids misbehave and don't pay attention, or you overreact to a little goofing off and rule with severe authority.

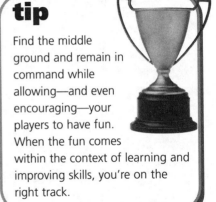

tip

Find the middle ground and remain in command while allowing—and even encouraging—your players to have fun. When the fun comes within the context of learning and improving skills, you're on the right track.

Be Dependable and Stable

Be on time at every practice and game, and be there ready to execute your plan. If you can't make a game or practice, alert your assistant coach or a parent who is willing and able to take over.

The kids are counting on you. When they know they can rely on you to be there and be ready, that lets them focus on learning, practicing, and performing. When the kids know that you respond evenly and fairly in all situations, they feel free to practice without worrying about how you might respond to a poor pass or a missed assignment on defense. Coaches who are dependable and stable create a healthy learning environment for their players.

Be Patient

If you're a parent, you know the value of patience. It can be difficult enough raising a couple of young kids. When you have 15 youngsters at your charge, patience is at a premium.

They won't pay attention to your every word. They won't always understand your instruction on the first, or second or third, try. They will make the same types of errors over and over again. They will ask you goofy questions and act, well, like the kids they are. They will, in short, try your patience. If you don't have a lot, here's your chance to develop this virtue.

Don't expect perfection, either in game time performance or practice field behavior. Let the kids know what you expect of them, in terms of their behavior and their listening to your directives. Also keep in mind what the goal is for the day, whether you're at a practice or a game, and steer the ship in that direction. When you guide your players with patient resolve, your practices will be more effective.

Don't mistake being patient with letting your players do whatever they want to do. Don't tolerate inappropriate words or actions. Step in and correct players in these situations. Just remember to be patient as they strive to learn how to dribble, pass, receive passes, shoot, and execute all the other skills involved in playing soccer.

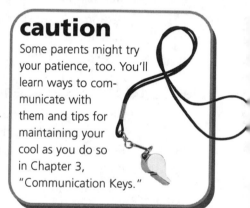

caution
Some parents might try your patience, too. You'll learn ways to communicate with them and tips for maintaining your cool as you do so in Chapter 3, "Communication Keys."

Be Flexible

Being flexible is another hallmark of a good coach. You might have worked out your season plan, in terms of what you want to teach and when you want to teach it, but you might have to adjust that schedule if the kids haven't picked up the requisite skills yet. For example, it's no use teaching your 10-year-olds how to execute a give-and-go if they haven't mastered the fundamentals of passing.

You have to constantly assess how your players are doing, what they need to learn next, and what they have been able to master at least well enough to move on to something new. It's good to work out a season plan in advance; just be ready to adjust that plan along the way.

Enjoy Getting to Know Your Players

Hopefully you enjoy being around kids, or you wouldn't have volunteered to coach. The best coaches appreciate kids for who they are and want to help them develop their skills and learn a sport. These coaches understand that their players are full-fledged children, not miniature adults. And these coaches enjoy being around their players. They can see the game from their players' perspectives while maintaining their adult view and their authority as a coach. They appreciate each child for his own unique personality and skills.

With that in mind, realize that the approach that works with Justin, who is effusive and outgoing, might not work with Sam, who is quiet and reflective. Learn to communicate with players on an individual level. Pay attention to what each player responds best to, and develop a rapport with each child that will help him learn and grow best.

That doesn't mean you should change your personality to suit each player. It means you should be aware of each child's distinct personality and relate to him as an individual.

Getting to know your players on an individual level is one of the joys of coaching. By doing so, you can tune into their needs as players and more readily help them develop their skills.

Desire to Help Kids Learn and Grow

After stopping an attack, a teammate passes to Susan, your goalkeeper, to clear the ball. Susan picks up the ball and prepares to punt it when she is whistled for a ball-handling violation. She didn't realize the goalkeeper can't field a ball with her hands when a teammate intentionally passes it to her.

Is this frustrating for you? Yes, especially if you've already told her this rule. You have two choices at this point:

- First, you could chew Susan out in front of the other players for her bone-headed play, shouting that you've gone over and over the goalkeeper rules with her and how she should know them by now, adding that she should have passed to Jonathon on her right side in the first place, rather than punt the ball.

- Second, you could calmly remind Susan of the rule and tell her the next time she's in that situation to pass the ball to a teammate. Then tell her to let it go, give her some sincere encouragement, and turn your attention back to the game.

Hopefully, you would choose the latter. You're more likely to do so if your focus is on helping the players learn and grow. This is really what coaching is all about at the youth level. It's very satisfying to watch your players acquire new skills, learn the game's tactics, and be able to execute plays more consistently. These things happen when your central desire as a coach is to help them learn and grow.

Be an Encourager

Good instruction is the seed and encouragement is the water that helps the seed grow. Your players need your encouragement as they attempt to learn the physical and mental skills it takes to play soccer. You'll learn more about specific ways to encourage your players in Chapter 3.

Be Willing to Learn

Just as your players will be learning throughout the season how to play the game, you'll be learning how to coach. There are many ways you can learn:

- **Through this book**—Use this guide to shape your approach to coaching and to formulate your season and practice plans.

- **Through your own experience**—Know that you'll make some mistakes along the way. That's okay. Be willing to learn from your mistakes. You'll discover, through experience, what works for you and what doesn't. You might also find that what works well for you this year might not work as well next year with different players.

- **Through observing other coaches**—You can learn from both good and bad coaches. What sets good coaches apart from ones who aren't so good? How do they communicate with their players, and *what* do they communicate? How do they behave on the sidelines? How do they relate with referees, and what kind of coaching do they do during the game? How do their players conduct themselves during and after the game? You can learn a lot through observation. Put to use what works for you, and model yourself after competent and caring coaches.

- **Through coaching clinics**—If your league offers a coaching clinic, attend it. If not, keep your eye out for coaching clinics in your area. You can often pick up some pointers and make helpful contacts at these clinics.

Most importantly, be willing to learn to coach. Many former players rely solely on their playing experience to inform their coaching. With that same thinking, you might assume that because you've had experience sitting in a dentist's chair and having a tooth drilled, you are qualified to pick up a dentist's drill and go to work in someone's mouth.

Playing and coaching call on a different set of skills. Having playing experience can help you as a coach in many ways, but it doesn't take the place of knowing how to coach. This book will help you develop your coaching skills.

Have a Sense of Humor

Enjoy your time as a coach. Soccer is meant to be fun. Your intent as a coach shouldn't be to "entertain the troops," but there's nothing wrong with a little natural levity. It's okay to laugh and joke with your players; you can do this while still moving forward with your instruction.

Just make sure your humor doesn't come at the expense of someone else—even an opponent. Don't make fun of someone's mistake, but do enjoy lighthearted moments as they come up.

caution

Having fun and being friendly with the kids doesn't mean you should try to be best buds with them. They're not looking for a new friend; they're looking for a coach to help them learn the game.

Don't use humor when kids need instruction, but do use it to diffuse tension. For example, if you are about to put Trevor into a game in which you're trailing by two goals with just a few minutes left, and he asks you what he should do, don't respond, "Why don't you score three goals? That would help us out tremendously." Trevor's not asking for a joke; he's asking for a little guidance. He'd be better-served if you told him, "Let's move the ball around. Look to attack their left side. They're weaker over there."

10 Keys to Being a Good Coach

We've just gone over the attributes of a good coach. If you have those attributes, or can develop them, you're on your way to being a good coach. But some other key elements to coaching extend beyond these basic characteristics. When you exhibit the traits we talked about in the previous section and possess the 10 keys we present in this section, you'll excel.

What are the keys to good coaching? To be a good soccer coach, you must

- Know the basics of the sport.
- Plan for your season and practices.
- Conduct effective practices.
- Teach skills and tactics.
- Correct players in a way that helps them improve.
- Teach and model good sporting behavior.
- Provide for safety.
- Communicate effectively with players, parents, referees, and league administrators.

■ Coach effectively during games.

■ Know what constitutes success in youth soccer.

Let's look at each of these keys in a little more depth.

Know the Basics of the Sport

You can't teach what you don't know. You need to be prepared to teach your players the basic rules, skills, and tactics of soccer. Especially at the younger ages, this information is quite basic, but that doesn't mean you automatically know all you need to know.

The next chapter covers the basic rules, and Chapters 9 and 10 cover the skills and tactics you need to know and teach. Be sure you know the rules, skills, and tactics before your season begins.

Plan for Your Season and Practices

You can know all you need to know about the rules, skills, and tactics, but if you don't have a game plan for when and how to teach them, you—and, more importantly, your players—will be in trouble.

Planning doesn't mean thinking about a drill you might run that day as you drive to practice. It means considering the big picture for the entire season and breaking that picture down into individual practice plans so you're prepared for every practice. You'll learn how to create season and practice plans in Chapter 5.

Conduct Effective Practices

When you have a practice plan in hand, you are on your way to conducting an effective practice. But, there's a big difference between having a plan and being able to execute it. Two coaches could have the exact same practice plan, and the experiences could be vastly different for their players depending on how the coaches execute that plan. In Chapter 5 you'll learn the keys to conducting effective practices.

Teach Skills and Tactics

This, of course, is one of your primary duties. Your ability to teach skills and tactics will significantly impact your players' development. Remember, the abilities to *perform* and to *teach* are different abilities. So, if you've played before, don't assume your playing experience will make you a great teacher.

Rather, learn how to be an effective teacher. In Chapter 6 you'll learn the keys to teaching skills and tactics.

Correct Players in a Way That Helps Them Improve

If one of your players makes the same mistake repeatedly, it might be he's simply unable to perform the skill yet—or it might be you haven't helped him understand *how* to correct his error. Part of being an effective teacher is being able to observe your players' performances, detect mechanical and tactical errors, and help them correct those errors. In Chapter 6, you'll learn how to detect and correct errors and help your players improve their skills.

Teach and Model Good Sporting Behavior

Your players will take their cues from you, not only on how to play the game, but also in how to behave at games. Behave responsibly and treat all involved with respect. You'll learn more on modeling good behavior in Chapter 7.

Provide for Players' Safety

This is one of your most important duties. You'll need to know how to conduct safe practices and how to respond to injuries when they occur. Chapter 4, "Safety Principles," is devoted to this topic.

Communicate Effectively

You'll do a lot of communicating as a coach, primarily with your players, but also with their parents, referees, other coaches, and league administrators. You might know exactly how to dribble, but if you don't know how to communicate how to do so, your players probably won't understand the mechanics involved. Chapter 3 explains how to communicate effectively—and what needs to be communicated and to whom—in a variety of situations.

Coach Effectively During Games

There's a difference between coaching at practice and coaching during games. The goals are different, and what you communicate is different. You'll learn about those differences, and the keys to coaching effectively during games, in Chapter 7.

Know What Success Is

By now you should have the idea that success at the youth level isn't based on your winning percentage. Rather, it's based on your ability to develop your players' skills and help them maintain their enthusiasm for the game, and on many other factors. Winning is an important and worthy goal, but you can have a successful season no matter what your record is. In Chapter 8, "Ingredients of a Successful Season," you'll learn what makes a season *truly* successful, and you'll also learn how to gauge your success.

Final Thoughts on the Keys to Being a Good Coach

When you use these 10 keys as the foundation of your coaching, you'll be successful. In fact, learning how to use these keys is what the rest of Part I, "Coaching Basics," is all about.

What to Expect As a Coach

The dream of youth league coaches goes something like this:

- All their players show up on time for every practice.
- The players pay attention every minute.
- The players soak in the instruction and acquire the physical skills and tactical knowledge with ease.
- The players perform like seasoned veterans from game 1.
- The parents are enthusiastic, supportive, and appreciative of the coach's efforts and ability to bring the team together.
- After winning the league championship, the players are somehow able to hoist the coach up on their scrawny shoulders and the parents roar their approval.
- To cap everything off, one rich parent throws a victory party at an expensive steak house, and during the party the teary-eyed parents come by, one by one, to thank the coach for making such a difference in their son's or daughter's life.

Conversely, the nightmare of youth league coaches goes something like this:

- You have to call all your players the night before the first practice because the league switched your practice field at the last moment.
- Not all the players assigned to your team show up for the first practice.
- The time you meant to take to plan for the season and the first practice evaporated, and you feel rushed and unprepared.
- About half the kids on your team have never played soccer before.
- A couple of kids are uncooperative.
- Another kid sprains his ankle in the first practice.
- At the first game, three of your starters show up late, so you have to rearrange everything at the last moment.
- You find that two fathers are more than willing to shout "helpful" coaching tips to you, while a mother sits in a lawn chair and critiques the referee throughout the game.
- After the game, a couple of parents complain about what position you played their child in, or what strategy you did (or didn't) employ.

- Heavy rains wipe out three games.
- Your calls to the league administrator are never returned.

Hopefully that nightmare won't be your reality. But the point is this: Be prepared for anything. Know that mundane, tedious, and sometimes bothersome things will infiltrate your season.

Expect to be tested—in some ways by your players, in others by their parents. Expect the refereeing to be less than perfect. Expect a few rainouts and a few hastily scheduled makeup dates at inopportune times. Expect your players to make mistakes, and expect some of them to be upset by those mistakes. Expect some parents to be very supportive, others to be seemingly nonexistent, and a few to present challenging situations. Expect the unexpected, and know that not all things will go according to your plan.

Keep your focus on what's best for the kids, and base all your decisions on that. That's why it's so important to develop the attributes of a good coach. When you are patient, flexible, dependable, and comfortable with being in charge, you can handle any situation that comes your way.

What Is Expected of *You* As a Coach

What is expected of you is summed up in the keys to good coaching:

- You are expected to know the basics of soccer, its rules, its strategies, and the skills involved.
- You are expected to be prepared to coach—to plan for the season and for practices—so that there is a logical cohesiveness to your instruction, a purpose for each practice, and a sense of moving forward throughout the season, with the players always learning and always improving.
- You are expected to be able to teach the skills and tactics of soccer, explain when and how each skill or tactic is used, and demonstrate how to execute it. (If you are unable to adequately demonstrate it, you can use an assistant coach or a volunteer parent to do so.)
- You are expected to observe your players as they practice the skills and tactics to detect what they are doing incorrectly and to help them make corrections.
- You are expected to model good sporting behavior; communicate appropriately with players, parents, referees, and the opposition; and show respect for all involved.
- You are expected to teach your players how to win with class without rubbing it in or taunting their opponents, and how to lose with dignity, learning from the loss and making neither a win nor a loss bigger than it is.

- You are expected to conduct practices as safely as possible, providing direct supervision at all times, conducting drills and games that are safe, warning players about inherent dangers, and instituting team rules that promote safety.

- You are expected to know how to coach during games, doing what's appropriate and best for your players' development and conducting yourself appropriately.

- Finally, you are expected to keep in mind what constitutes success in youth soccer. You are striving to win your games, of course, but far greater than that, you are giving your players opportunities to develop their skills, to have fun, to compete, to play together as a team, and to get the most of their abilities. They are there to grow, learn, and develop, and that development is your main task.

Now, not all parents or players will have these expectations. Some will be focused only on winning and become frustrated if your coaching decisions don't reflect the same outlook. In Chapter 3 you'll learn when and how to communicate with players and parents who have these expectations.

It's important that you keep these expectations in mind throughout the season. They will act as your rudder, guiding you through any choppy waters you might experience.

Equipment and Insurance

Check with your league regarding equipment they issue each team and insurance they might carry. In some cases, the league provides soccer balls, cones, and other equipment for coaches. It's your responsibility to keep and maintain the equipment and return it at season's end.

In some cases, insurance is provided through a coaching certification program or a league; in other cases, it's not provided. Some leagues carry insurance policies that cover all teams and participants involved, including coaches and referees. If insurance is an important issue to you, talk to your league administrator about it.

Last, But Not Least: Why Kids Play Soccer

Kids play soccer for a lot of reasons. Some have grand dreams of being the next Mia Hamm, Brandi Chastain, Claudio Reyna, Brian McBride, or whoever their favorite player is.

Some play for negative reasons, such as their parents pushing them into it. Or, they might have chosen soccer over a less desirable activity, such as taking tuba lessons.

But the overwhelming majority play for positive reasons. Those reasons are

- They want to have fun.
- They want to hang out with their friends.

- They want to develop their abilities.
- They like the excitement of sports.
- They want to be part of a winning effort.

That order is not random; it reflects the most common responses kids give when they are asked for the main reasons they play soccer.

Notice that *fun* is at the top of the list and *winning* is at the bottom. Winning is important to them, but not nearly as important as it is to have fun and be with their friends.

What does this mean for you? It means you should focus on fun and development throughout the season and that you should strive to win, but not at the expense of fun and development. It's that simple. And you'll be amazed at how well your players perform when they're having fun and developing their skills.

THE ABSOLUTE MINIMUM

This chapter introduced you to the basic concepts of coaching soccer. You learned about your coaching approach, the attributes of a good coach, the keys to being a good coach, what you should expect as a coach, what is expected of you as a coach, and why kids play soccer. Keep these points in mind:

- Base your coaching approach on players' fun and development. Always keep their overall development in mind.
- Keep the attributes of a good coach front and center. When you approach your coaching with these traits in mind, you are bound to be successful.
- Plan your practices. Learn how to teach skills and tactics and how to correct mistakes.
- Expect the unexpected, and be guided by your coaching approach in all situations.
- Live up to your own expectations, based on the keys to good coaching.
- Understand that kids play soccer to have fun, to be with their friends, and to develop their skills.

Coaching with these things in mind will help you plan and implement a fun and constructive soccer season that produces enjoyment and plenty of learning!

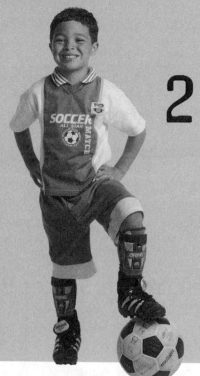

2

RULES OF THE GAME

Soccer has some basic rules that even the most casual fan knows:

- Only the goalie can touch the ball with her hands.
- Kick (or head) the ball in the goal and you score.
- Play resumes with a throw-in when a player kicks the ball beyond the sideline.
- You can't trip, hold, or push an opponent.

There are many rules beyond these that your players need to know, and as their coach, it's your duty to teach them those rules. What's a corner kick, and when does it happen? What's the difference between a direct free kick and an indirect free kick? What's a penalty kick, and when is it awarded? What's a goal kick, and what are the rules concerning it?

The rules for youth soccer are derived from the 17 *laws* of the sport. (Throughout this book, I refer to these laws as *rules* because the latter term is more commonly recognized by most Americans, especially those who are only vaguely familiar with the sport.) These rules are modified to make the sport appropriate for various levels of youth play: U-6 (under 6 years old), U-8, U-10, and so on. Common modifications include field size, ball size, game length, the number of players on the field, how players can be substituted, how fouls are handled, and so on. Check with your league administrator to learn which modified rules your league has in place.

In this chapter, then, you'll learn about the basic rules so you can prepare your players to know how to operate on both offense and defense.

Basic Youth Soccer Rules

The following is meant to be a primer for the basics, not the final word on every rule in complete detail. The rules in this section are divided into these categories:

- Field
- Equipment
- Game length
- Players
- Starts and restarts
- Moving the ball
- Fouls
- Offside
- Goalkeeping
- Scoring
- Officials

Field

Soccer is played on a rectangular field that differs in length and width according to age level and field availability. A regulation adult field is somewhere between 100 and 130 yards long and 50–100 yards wide, but for youth play those dimensions are somewhere around half that size. See Figure 2.1 for a depiction of a field.

Equipment

Soccer is played with a size 3 or 4 ball, depending on league rules for age levels. Usually, U-6 and U-8 use a size 3 and U-10 and U-12 use a size 4.

FIGURE 2.1

A soccer field.

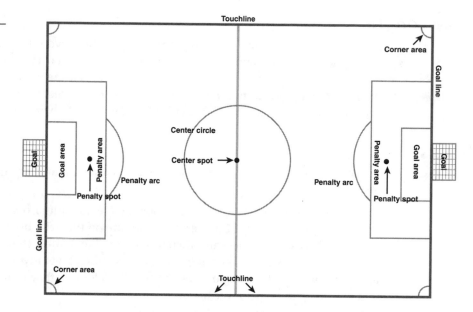

Players wear rubber-cleated shoes (tennis shoes are fine for younger kids) and shin guards under knee-length socks (see Figure 2.2). It's best if they wear loose-fitting clothing to allow freedom of movement. In addition, goalkeepers often wear protective gloves (see Figure 2.3). Goalies can also wear elbow and knee pads for additional protection. Jewelry, such as watches, necklaces, bracelets, and similar items, isn't allowed because it puts players in danger of being injured.

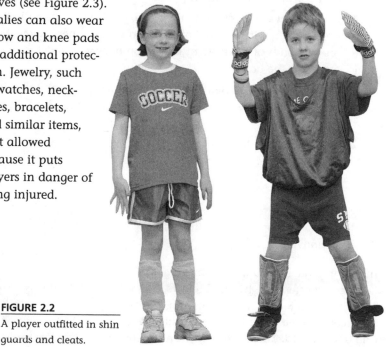

FIGURE 2.2

A player outfitted in shin guards and cleats.

FIGURE 2.3

A goalkeeper with protective gloves.

Game Length

Leagues devise game lengths according to the ages of the players. In the adult version, a regulation game comprises two 45-minute halves with a 15-minute intermission; in youth play, younger players might play four 10-minute quarters and older children might play two 25-minute halves. Check with your league on how long your games are and whether they're divided in quarters or halves.

Players

In this section, we talk about the number of players allowed, player positions, and substitution rules.

The number of players allowed on the field for each team varies from league to league. In traditional soccer, 11 players per team are on the field, but most youth leagues play short-sided games, anywhere from 8-on-8 to 3-on-3. These short-sided games provide players more touches of the ball, increase player involvement, and reduce the chances of clustering around the ball. In addition, they foster skill development because players get more action.

Player positions include the following:

- **Forwards**—Tend to shoot more often than other players. Those who play nearer the sidelines are called *wingers*, and those who play near the middle of the field are called *strikers*.

- **Midfielders**—Are closer to their own goalkeeper than the forwards are. They often get in on more of the action than other players because they play on both ends of the field, attacking on offense and defending when the other team has the ball.

- **Defenders**—Are closer to their own goalkeeper than the midfielders are. They often initiate the offensive attack and remain back to defend against a counterattack.

- **Goalkeeper**—Defends the goal. He is the only player who can use his hands. He can catch the ball, deflect it with his hands, and use any part of his body to keep the ball out of the goal. He also initiates the offense from within the penalty area.

In a 6-on-6 game, you might have a goalkeeper, two defenders, two midfielders, and one forward; in an 8-on-8 game, you might have a goalkeeper, three defenders, three midfielders, and one forward. There are many formations you can use; these are just examples of a few you might employ.

note

There's great fluidity of movement in soccer, and players other than the goalkeeper shouldn't feel locked into staying in one location. One way to approach positions is to coach your players to generally remain on the left side or right side of the field (whichever side they began on).

Check your league for substitution rules. Some leagues stipulate the number of substitutions that can be made during a game, and some allow an unlimited number of substitutes. Some leagues allow substitutes to enter a game as play continues (with the player she is replacing leaving the game at the same time); other leagues require play to be stopped before a substitute can come onto the field.

Starts and Restarts

A game starts with a kickoff. If the ball goes out of bounds, play restarts with a throw-in, goal kick, or corner kick, depending on how the ball went out. In this section we consider all four ways of starting and restarting play.

Kickoff

A *kickoff* is used to start a game, to start the second half and to restart play after a goal. The referee places the ball in the center circle, and the kicker must kick the ball into the opposing half of the field (that is, toward the opponents' goal). All opposing players must be outside the center circle, and all players must be on their own side of the field until the ball is kicked. The ball is required to move forward before another player can play it. The kicker can't touch the ball after he has kicked it until another player has touched it.

If you are playing by halves, the team that didn't kick off to begin the first half gets to kick off to begin the second half. The team that is scored upon gets to kick off after a goal.

Throw-in

When the ball goes out of bounds on a sideline, it is put back in play with a *throw-in*. The team that did not touch the ball last before it went out of bounds throws it in. Note that the ball has to completely cross the sideline before it is considered out of bounds. A ball on the line is not out.

tip

Some players seem more naturally suited to being forwards—they're stronger-legged, have better ball-handling skills, and have more accurate shooting skills. Others might enjoy playing defense more, and some players might gravitate toward goalkeeping. All of this is fine; play these players in the positions they excel in. But at younger levels, let players play in different positions. As they reach age 10, they can begin to specialize in one position.

note

Usually the player kicking off kicks the ball so that a teammate can play it, rather than kicking the ball deep into the opponents' territory.

A throw-in is the only time a player other than the goalkeeper can intentionally touch the ball with her hands.

On a throw-in, the player must use two hands on the ball, bringing it above and behind her head before throwing it (see Figure 2.4). Both feet must be on the ground at the time of the release, and the player throwing it in cannot touch the ball again until another player has touched it.

Goal Kick

A *goal kick* is taken by the defense when the offense kicks the ball out of bounds beyond the *goal line* (the end line that runs the width of the field). Any player on the defense can take the goal kick, kicking the ball from anywhere inside the goal area (see Figure 2.5). The opposing team cannot be in the penalty area when the kick is taken. The kicker cannot play the ball again until another player has touched it, and the ball is not considered in play until it travels beyond the penalty area.

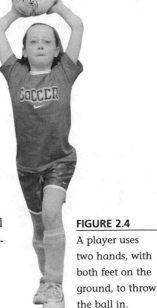

FIGURE 2.4

A player uses two hands, with both feet on the ground, to throw the ball in.

FIGURE 2.5

A goal kick.

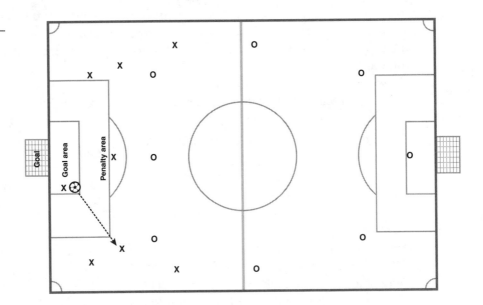

X – players on team making goal kick

O – players on team defending against goal kick

⊛ – ball

----- pass

Corner Kick

A *corner kick* is the flip side of a goal kick. In this case, the ball has gone out of bounds beyond a goal line, but it's the defense that has sent the ball out of bounds. The offense puts the ball in play with a corner kick. One player kicks the ball from the corner of the field closest to where the ball went out. Defenders can't be within 3–10 yards of the player making the corner kick (the distance depends on the size of the field), but offensive players can position themselves wherever they want. Once the ball is in play, the corner kicker can't touch the ball until another player has played it. A goal can be scored directly on a corner kick. See Figure 2.6 for a corner kick.

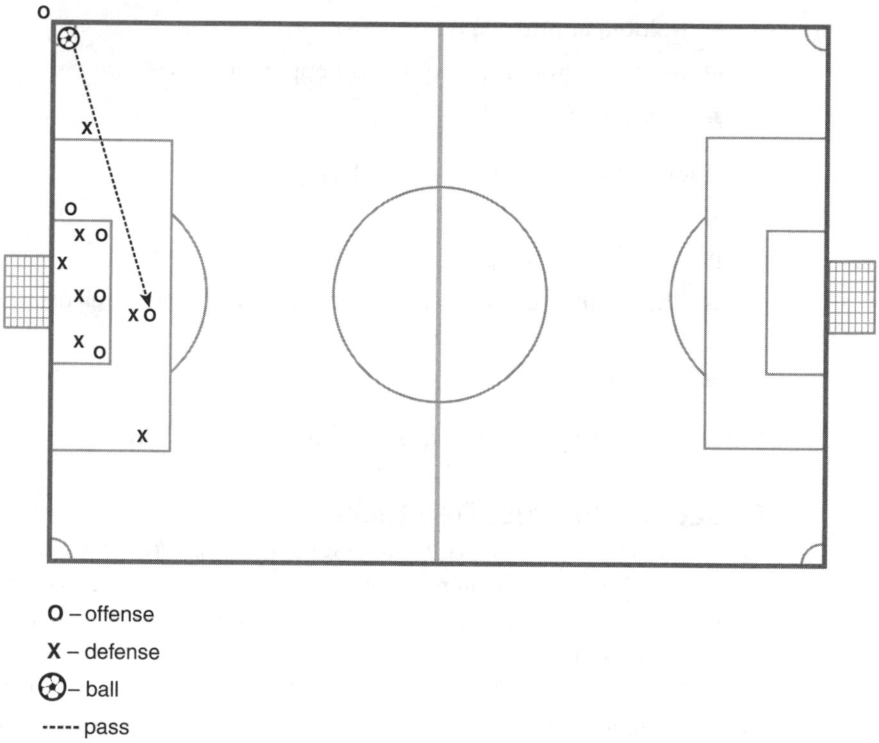

FIGURE 2.6

A corner kick.

O – offense
X – defense
⊛ – ball
----- pass

Moving the Ball

In most countries, soccer is known as *football*—for good reason. The way to move the ball is with the feet. Players can dribble the ball (maintain possession as they move with the ball, kicking it a short distance) or pass the ball by kicking it to a teammate.

Except for the goalie and a player executing a throw-in, players cannot touch the ball with their hands or arms. If the referee judges that the touch with a hand or arm is unintentional—as in the ball is kicked into the player's arm—no foul is committed. If the touch is intentional, the referee calls a foul and gives the ball to the other team.

Fouls

The referee calls a foul for a number of actions. Play stops with the referee's whistle. After he signals the foul, the ball is put back in play with a direct free kick, an indirect free kick, or a penalty kick, depending on the type of foul and where it occurred.

The following fouls result in a direct free kick (the types of kicks will be explained in a moment):

- Handball
- Kicking, striking, or tripping an opponent
- Holding or pushing an opponent
- Jumping at or charging into an opponent
- Charging from behind

These fouls result in an indirect free kick:

- Playing dangerously
- Obstructing an opponent
- The goalkeeper taking more than 6 seconds before releasing possession of the ball with his hands
- Offside

Following are descriptions of free kicks and penalty kicks.

Direct and Indirect Free Kicks

When the referee makes a call that results in a *direct free kick*, the kick is taken from the spot of the foul. Any member of the team that was fouled can take the kick. The opposing team must be at least 3–10 yards away from the ball until it is kicked (again, the distance depends on the size of the field. The only exception here is if the kick comes within 10 yards of the opponents' goal; the opponents have the right to defend their goal, even if they are closer than 10 yards from the ball.

The player taking the kick can score directly; the ball doesn't have to touch another player first.

An *indirect kick* is administered the same as a direct free kick, but the kicker cannot score directly on the play. The ball must be touched by another player before a goal can be scored.

Penalty Kick

The referee issues a *penalty kick* when a defender commits a violation within her own penalty area that calls for a direct free kick. The referee places the ball on the penalty spot, normally 12 yards away from the goal (though some leagues might place the penalty spot closer to the goal for younger players), and the kicker kicks the ball from that spot, attempting to score, while the goalkeeper defends the goal (see Figure 2.7). The goalie can move sideways before the kick, but he cannot move forward until the kick is taken. All other players must be out of the penalty area.

FIGURE 2.7

A penalty kick.

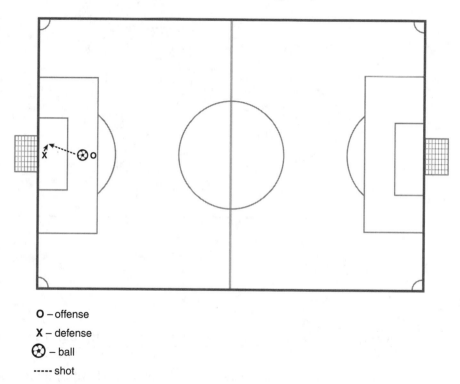

O – offense

X – defense

⊗ – ball

----- shot

If the goalkeeper stops the ball and it rebounds into the field, play continues unabated. Likewise, if the goalkeeper catches the kick, he puts the ball into play as he normally does after stopping a kick. If the ball goes out of bounds after being touched by the goalkeeper, the opposing team puts the ball into play with a corner kick.

Offside

Offside is a rule that prevents a team from having one or more players hang around the opponents' goal. A player is offside if there is only one defensive player (including the goalkeeper) between himself and the goal (see Figure 2.8). If two defensive players, including the goalie, are between the offensive player and the goal, the player is not offside. When offside is called, the opposing team gets an indirect free kick at the spot of the infraction.

FIGURE 2.8

An offside infraction.

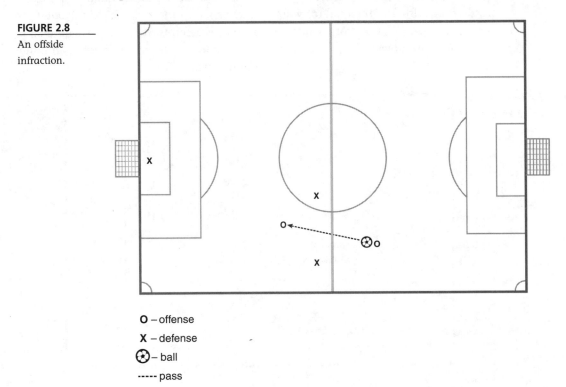

O – offense
X – defense
⊗ – ball
----- pass

A player can't be offside, regardless of defensive positioning, if she is on her end of the field (that is, closer to her own goal than to the opponents').

Many youth leagues have relaxed offside rules; check with your league administrator so you know how to instruct your players here.

Goalkeeping

Because the goalkeeper is the only player who can use his hands (other than players making a throw-in), the goalie often wears a different-colored shirt. This helps the referee easily distinguish him.

These rules pertain to goalkeepers:

- They *can* use their hands within the goal area but not beyond it.
- They *can* use their hands to field a ball that a teammate has intentionally kneed or headed to them.
- They *cannot* use their hands to field a ball that a teammate has intentionally kicked to them.
- They *cannot* use their hands to pick up a throw-in from a teammate.
- They *cannot* touch the ball with their hands after they release it from their possession until another player touches it.

> **note** 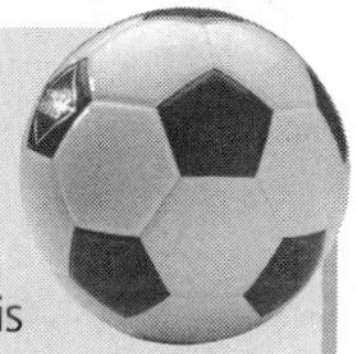
>
> A player is not ruled offside if he is in an offside position but is not participating in the play. If the play is taking place on the other side of the field, and the player in the offside position is not involved, the player is not offside. The reasoning here is the player's team has not gained an advantage from the player's offside positioning.

Goalkeepers can distribute the ball to their teammates by rolling it, throwing it, or kicking it. You'll learn about these skills in Chapter 10, "Defensive Skills and Tactics."

Scoring

A goal is scored when the ball passes fully beyond the goal line and into the goal. A team can't score a goal directly from a throw-in or an indirect free kick; on these plays the ball must be touched by at least one other player besides the kicker before a goal counts.

Officials

Figures 2.9a–i show the signals referees make as they officiate a soccer game. Note that many volunteer referees aren't used to signaling and haven't been trained to use signals. If you're unclear of a call, ask the referee to clarify the call.

FIGURE 2.9A–I

Referee signals: (a) Goal (pointing to the center of the field to restart); (b) Penalty kick (pointing to penalty area); (c) Corner kick (pointing to the corner area); (d) Goal kick (pointing to the goal area); (e) Advantage or play on; (f) Offside (the assistant referee holds up a flag; the referee points to the spot of the infraction); (g) Indirect free kick; (h) Direct free kick; (i) Caution or ejection.

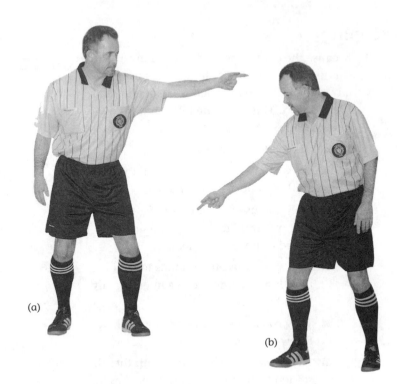

(a)

(b)

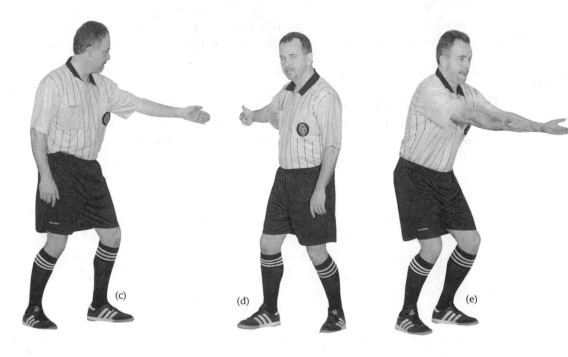

(c)

(d)

(e)

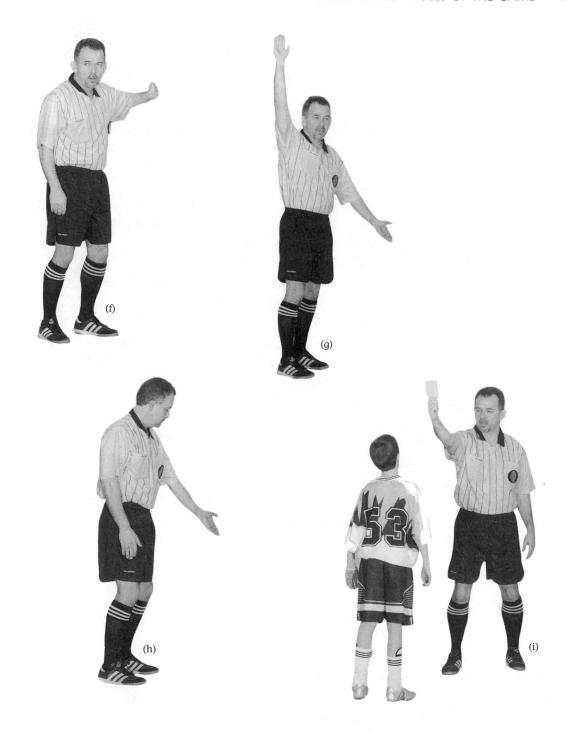

(f)

(g)

(h)

(i)

Terms

Following are some soccer terms that will help you understand the game and its rules:

- **Advantage or play on**—This refers to a referee seeing a foul committed by the defense but not calling it (refer to Figure 2.9e). When would a referee not call a foul? He wouldn't if doing so would give an advantage to the defense, or if the offense would lose the advantage it was maintaining even though the foul occurred.

- **Charge**—A defensive player is assessed a charging foul when he uses body contact to cause an offensive player to lose possession of the ball.

- **Dribbling**—This skill allows a player to maintain possession of the ball, while moving, by kicking it close by.

- **Encroachment**—This occurs when a defender advances within 10 yards of the ball before a player takes a free kick.

- **Foul**—A foul is a rule infraction for which a penalty is prescribed.

- **Free kick**—The ball is put back into play with a free kick after a foul has occurred. Depending on the foul, the team fouled puts the ball into play with a direct free kick or an indirect free kick.

- **Goal area**—This is the area immediately around the goal. The goalkeeper can use his hands in this area.

- **Goal line**—This is the line that extends the width of the field.

- **Live ball**—This means the ball is in play.

- **Pass**—This refers to one player passing or moving the ball to another player, using any body part other than the hands. (The goalkeeper can pass the ball using his hands.)

- **Penalty area**—This is the area in front of the goal in which a penalty kick is taken.

- **Tackle**—This refers to a defender taking the ball away from the player in control of it.

- **Touchlines**—These are the sidelines on the field. The entire line is within the field of play.

- **Warning**—This is a verbal admonition to a coach or player for poor conduct. Repeat warnings can result in ejection.

Now let's move to some different subjects: your own learning process as a coach and the process of teaching rules to your players.

Keep on Learning

Knowing the rules is one of your primary duties because it influences how you coach and instruct your players and which strategies you use during a game. So, know the rules, impart them to your players, and coach accordingly.

You can find more in-depth information on soccer rules on various websites and from youth soccer organizations.

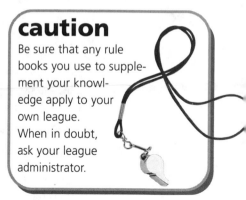

caution

Be sure that any rule books you use to supplement your knowledge apply to your own league. When in doubt, ask your league administrator.

Teaching Rules to Your Players

To help your players know the rules, you need to know three things, in this order:

1. What your players *need* to know

2. What they *do* know

3. How to best impart what your players need to learn

Your players need to know the basics: what constitutes a foul; when and how direct free kicks, indirect free kicks, and penalty kicks are taken; what offside is and how to avoid it, if it is called in your league; when and how kickoffs, goal kicks, corner kicks, and throw-ins are executed; and what the goalkeeper can and cannot do.

As you begin practicing and place your kids in game situations, it will become evident which rules they know and which rules they don't know. At that point, it's up to you to make sure they learn what they need.

How should you go about teaching rules? Doing your best imitation of a classroom lecturer is definitely *not* the best way. Here are four ways you can help your players learn the rules of soccer:

- Situational plays
- Practice games
- Brief discussions
- Players' experiences

Let's take a look at each way.

Situational Plays

If you want your players to learn how to execute (and defend against) corner kicks, goal kicks, penalty kicks, and free kicks, put them in those situations and let them learn. See how much they understand, and fill in the gaps or correct their misconceptions about what they can and can't do.

Practice Games

You can also use scrimmages to see how much your players know and how they respond to various situations, and to teach them the correct response when they're unclear on what they should do. In this setting, your teaching focus is broader: You provide instruction in whatever area you see your players need it. In one moment, in terms of rules understanding, it might be on what constitutes a foul; in another, it might be how to proceed with a penalty kick or throw-in.

> **note**
>
> The primary focus on practice should be on developing the skills and tactical understanding it takes to make the plays individually and as a team. Look to slip in rules instruction within this skill instruction and practice.

When you use scrimmages in this manner, you have a couple of choices: You can briefly stop play and instruct your players as the need arises, or you can note what you need to tell them and then discuss your point(s) at the end of practice. In general, don't disrupt the flow of action unless it has broken down because the players need further skill or rules instruction.

Brief Discussions

The end-of-practice discussion is also a good time to briefly teach or remind players of a rule (or anything else important) that they appeared to have difficulty understanding in that practice.

For example, you might say, "I noticed that sometimes we're forgetting about the offside rule. Who can tell me what the offside rule is?" Ideally, at least a few players will be able to explain the rule. If a player offers a correct answer, repeat it for everyone to hear. If no one responds correctly, tell them what it means to be offside and make a note to work on that situation during the next practice.

> **tip**
>
> Offering praise for correct answers encourages players to respond to future questions. Never belittle players for incorrect answers. It makes your players feel bad, and they will be less likely to participate in other team discussions.

Use these practice-ending discussions to briefly make a point, ideally one that ties in directly to the activities of that practice. Don't drone on about various rules, especially if they don't relate to what the kids experienced that day. Kids learn better when the learning is practical and in context with what they're doing.

> **note**
>
> In the next chapter you'll learn effective ways to communicate with your players, both during practice and in end-of-practice discussions.

Players' Experiences

Imagine the coach that teaches his players the rules by the book. He sits them down in orderly rows; lectures them for 50 minutes; and then gives them a written test, which they all ace. (I told you you'd have to use your imagination.)

Then the first game arrives, and the players have no idea what the offside rule is, or why the referee blew his whistle when they held an opponent, or why the referee told them to move farther away from the opponent taking the free kick.

Book knowledge can't take the place of firsthand experience. Players learn rules best when they see them applied in the practices and games they play in, especially when they are involved in the plays. *Then* the rules begin to register.

And that's good news, because it means you don't have to spend your time lecturing to them about all the rules. You just instruct along the way, as they play. And everyone—yourself included—has more fun that way.

Part of your job as coach is to reinforce your players' learning from practice to practice and game to game. As you observe their performances and discover what they need to learn, you can teach them not only the skills of soccer, but also the rules.

The Absolute Minimum

This chapter focused on the basic rules of soccer. In addition, it provided terms that are helpful to know, refereeing signals, and ways to help your players learn. Points to keep in mind include

- You need to know not only the basic rules of soccer, but also any specific modifications your league has in place.

- Your players need to know the basic rules, and part of your responsibility is to determine what they do know and what they need to learn.

- After you know what your players need to learn, plan for effective ways to teach them the rules. These ways include using situational plays in practice, using scrimmages as teaching tools, holding brief end-of-practice discussions, and reinforcing players' learning through their own experiences gained during practices and games.

- You can expand your own knowledge of the rules by finding resources through your own league, through youth soccer organizations, and through resources you can find in your library or on the Web.

Your players need to know the rules to compete in games, but coaches often don't teach rules because they're so focused on teaching skills. You'll be a step ahead if you take the time to also teach your players the rules they need to know.

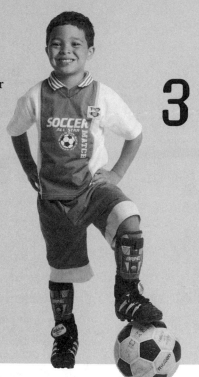

3

COMMUNICATION KEYS

As a coach, you're called on to do a lot of communicating. You address players, parents, other coaches, league administrators, and referees. You communicate in person, on the phone, in writing, one on one, and within group settings. How well you communicate with these groups significantly influences how successful your season is, how enjoyable it is, and how much your players learn.

Of course, you've been communicating all your life. It can't be that hard, right?

Right and wrong. If you haven't coached or taught before and aren't used to instructing and leading youngsters, then you are entering uncharted territory.

Consider this chapter your roadmap to help you chart that territory.

The 10 keys, presented first, will help you hone your communication skills as a coach. These keys are written with players in mind, but they apply to all groups you will communicate with. Following the keys, we'll focus on the specifics of communicating with parents, league administrators, opponents, and referees.

10 Keys to Being a Good Communicator

Most people tend to think only of the verbal side of communication. That's important, but there's so much more to being a good communicator. Here are 10 keys to good communication:

1. Know your message.
2. Make sure you are understood.
3. Deliver your message in the proper context.
4. Use appropriate emotions and tones.
5. Adopt a healthy communication style.
6. Be receptive.
7. Provide helpful feedback.
8. Be a good nonverbal communicator.
9. Be consistent.
10. Be positive.

Know Your Message

Coach Caravelli gathers his players at the practice field and says, "Alright, guys, today we're going to learn how to dribble." He kicks a ball several yards in front of him, runs after it, kicks it several yards in front again, and stops. "You want to push the ball out in front of you in the direction you want to go. It's that simple," he says.

"But Coach, my dad says you're supposed to keep the ball closer to you, or it will get stolen," one player says.

Coach Caravelli considers this a moment before saying, "Actually, let's just focus on passing today. Passing is a better way to move the ball. It's much quicker than dribbling."

The player was right; Coach Caravelli didn't know the technique for dribbling (which you'll learn in Chapter 9). He didn't really know his message.

Three issues are involved in knowing your message. You need to

■ Know the skills and rules you need to teach.

■ Read situations and respond appropriately.

■ Provide accurate and clear information.

Know the Skills and Rules

Coach Caravelli didn't know how to teach the skill of dribbling. He might be a smooth, coherent, and clear speaker, but that's not going to help his players learn how to dribble. Smoothness doesn't make up for lack of knowledge. You have to know the skills and rules.

Read the Situation

As Coach Caravelli teaches his players how to correctly execute a give-and-go play, Kenny and Sam are quietly goofing off, not paying attention. But Coach Caravelli doesn't address the situation because they're not really disrupting his instruction and he's a little behind schedule. As his players begin to practice give-and-gos, Kenny and Sam are not executing as instructed. They are not *going* after they *give*.

So, Coach Caravelli stops the action and tells them how to properly execute a give-and-go. Then he lets them proceed.

Coach Caravelli delivered an important part of the message—Kenny and Sam need to know how to execute a give-and-go—but that was only part of the message he should have delivered. The real issue here was that the players weren't paying attention, and Coach Caravelli didn't correct that situation when it was occurring. He should have corrected that on the spot. Barring that, he should have told Kenny and Sam that the reason they didn't know how to execute a give-and-go was because they weren't listening when he was teaching how to do so and that they need to listen to his instruction the first time around.

Sometimes knowing your message goes beyond understanding the content. You have to read the situation as well and tailor your message accordingly.

> **note**
>
> Eloquently stating and aptly showing how to perform a skill doesn't mean you're a good communicator if you can't keep your players' attention.

Provide Accurate and Clear Information

Knowing the content of your message isn't enough. You need to be able to deliver that content clearly and accurately.

Imagine a portion of a coach's preseason letter to parents reading like this:

> "I'm really looking forward to coaching your child this season. Our first practice is next Monday at 6 p.m. Please make sure your child remembers to wear shin guards!"

Too bad the coach didn't remember to note *where* the first practice is being held. As a result of not being clear in his letter, he'll have to spend a lot of time on the phone calling parents to deliver the information.

The same goes for teaching skills. Perhaps you know the proper technique for tackling, but your instruction is so technical and confusing that your players are worse off than if they'd received no instruction at all! They're confused, you're frustrated, and no one learns how to tackle.

Know what information you need to deliver, and deliver it clearly so that all concerned understand. That's sometimes easier said than done.

Make Sure You Are Understood

As you can imagine, if you are not clear with your directives, you can create a lot of confusion. Take the following example:

> "Okay, Dion," Coach Hagan says, "the next time you're in that situation, give a little half-volley with the side of your foot. Alan was open to your right, but by the time you got him the ball, he was covered."

Dion gives Coach Hagan a puzzled look, but Coach Hagan, in the midst of conducting a drill, doesn't notice. He's already preparing to set up the next play. Dion just hopes that same situation doesn't come again because he has no idea what a "half-volley" is.

Just because something is clear to you doesn't mean it's clear to whomever you're delivering your message to, be it a player, a parent, an administrator, or anyone else. You need to watch for understanding and be ready to clarify your message if the person on the receiving end is confused.

When you state your message clearly and simply, you increase your chances of being understood. But don't count on that; instead, watch your players' facial expressions and read their body language. If they look confused or unsure of what to do, state your instruction again, making sure you use language they understand.

And watch how you say things: When you encourage a goalie to "cut off the shooting angle," she might not understand what you mean. If she looks confused, tell her what the shooting angle is and how to move to lessen the angle.

Speak in language your players understand, and watch for their understanding.

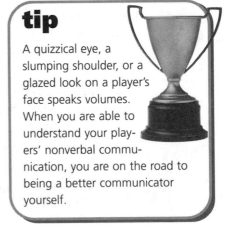

tip

A quizzical eye, a slumping shoulder, or a glazed look on a player's face speaks volumes. When you are able to understand your players' nonverbal communication, you are on the road to being a better communicator yourself.

Deliver Your Message in the Proper Context

Karim tackles the ball from an opponent and then begins to dribble downfield, keeping his head down. His progress is slow, but he does maintain control of the ball. Zach, his teammate, breaks free downfield and is in good position to receive a pass from Karim, but Karim is too focused on the ball. The potential to gain an advantage is lost, and eventually the ball is stolen from Karim. On the sideline, Coach Grantham cups his hands to his mouth:

> "Hey, Karim, you've got to see the field! Zach was wide open! Keep your head up when you dribble, like this!" Coach Grantham models keeping his head up as he dribbles a phantom ball a little ways down the sideline."

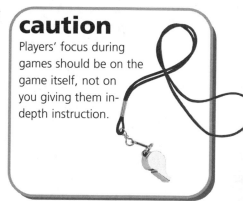

caution

Players' focus during games should be on the game itself, not on you giving them in-depth instruction.

What's wrong with this? First, it's humiliating for Karim to have everyone at the field witness his coach yelling at him and instructing him on how to dribble. Second, it's not the time or place to give detailed instruction. That should be done in practice, not in games. The instruction itself wasn't incorrect; the timing of it was.

So, consider your context for delivering your message. Give brief reminders of tactical or skill execution during games, but save the teaching for practices.

Use Appropriate Emotions and Tones

Emotions are a natural part of soccer. Both you and your players (and their parents) can expect to experience a range of emotions throughout the season. In terms of communicating with others, your emotions can significantly affect your message.

How? Let's look at a few examples:

> *Situation:* An opponent, while dribbling, lets the ball get too far in front of him, but Caitlyn simply maintains her position between the ball and the goal and doesn't make the tackle, which she easily could have done. As a result, the opponent regains control, passes, and his teammate scores.
>
> *Response #1:* "Come on, Caitlyn! You need to be more aggressive! Go after that ball! That should have been yours!"
>
> *Response #2:* "That's okay, guys! Let's move it up quickly. Be aggressive now."

Don't ever berate a player, publicly or privately. Remember that even Major League Soccer players make errors. Your players are going to make errors; what they need is instruction, if they're not sure what to do, and encouragement regardless. Help them to keep their focus on the game, not on how well they're pleasing you.

Situation: You are moments away from beginning the game that will decide your league championship.

Response #1: "This is it, guys! There's no tomorrow. We've been playing to get to this game all year long. Show them what you're made of. I want to feel that championship trophy in my hands at the end of the game. How about you? Are you ready to go out and win?"

Response #2: "Let's play soccer like we know how. Keep your focus on the fundamentals. Spread out the attack, make good passes, and keep the ball out of the danger zone on defense. Let's go out and have some fun, all right?"

Pep talks are better saved for the movies. Such talks often backfire because they get kids so sky high that they can't perform well. Your players need to focus on playing sound, fundamental soccer. Remind them of that and tell them to have fun.

Situation: In a scrimmage, Terrell keeps missing tackle attempts, letting his opponent slip by him as he goes for the ball.

Response #1: "Hey, Terrell, where are you going? Don't you know you're not supposed to run downfield unless your team has the ball?"

Response #2: "Don't overextend on the tackle, Terrell. Get in better position before you go for the ball. Until then, just mark the dribbler, okay? You can do it."

Sarcasm will get you nowhere. Terrell doesn't need sarcasm, or any type of humor. He needs instruction and encouragement.

Adopt a Healthy Communication Style

A lot of what you've been reading has to do with your communication style—whether you over-coach during games, offering too much instruction; whether you keep your emotions in check, or are too excitable or high-strung; what your tone is as you communicate; and so on. But there is more to consider concerning your communication style. It has to do with the bigger picture, with how you communicate on a daily basis. It has more to do with personality, outlook, and attitude than with reacting to a specific moment. And some styles are more effective than others.

Here are a few of the less-effective styles some coaches fall into:

- **Always talking, never listening**—Some coaches feel if they're not constantly talking, they're not providing the proper instruction their players need. Carried to the extreme, some feel that their players have nothing to say. Coaches who always talk and never listen tend to have players who stand around more in practice because their coach is talking, and those coaches don't get to know their players, thus missing out on one of the real joys of coaching soccer. *Deliver the messages you need to deliver, but don't feel you have to be talking throughout the entire practice.*

- **Always in control, too directive**—Some coaches run practices like drill sergeants, snapping orders at players, exerting their authority, and squelching fun wherever it begins to appear. When practice doesn't go exactly as they have choreographed it, they become irked. When players don't progress according to schedule, it drives them crazy. *Be in control of practice, yes, but don't squelch the fun and don't obsess over things you can't control.*

- **Not in control, too passive**—Other coaches take the opposite tack, either because they're unsure of themselves or they're too laid-back and give the impression that *no* one is in charge. They don't provide the guidance or discipline players need. Not comfortable in the spotlight, they avoid it, and discipline problems begin to crop up. *If you're a quiet or laid-back person, don't change your personality but do exert your authority as coach. You can be in charge and provide instruction without being loud and obnoxious.*

- **Seeking perfection**—There's a fine line between seeking to improve and seeking perfection. When coaches cross over the line into perfectionism, they are rarely satisfied with anything. Their players mark well, but they don't tackle to the coaches' satisfaction. They maintain control as they dribble, but they don't go fast enough. They pass well, but their receiving skills are average. Even the fields are not manicured to these coaches' satisfaction. Players are on edge when they play for a perfectionist coach; their focus turns from playing the game to pleasing the coach. *Help your players improve their skills, but allow them margin for error. You can strive for improvement without putting added stress on the kids. Celebrate improvement even if it's still not picture-perfect.*

- **Not in control of emotions**—Some coaches throw up their hands in frustration when players are trying hard but having difficulty learning a skill. They shout in anger at a questionable call made by a volunteer referee. Their voices drip with sarcasm when players ask them something they feel the players should know. They respond with overzealous enthusiasm when their team scores a goal in a tight game, and this response is seen by all as unsporting behavior. *The point is not to suppress all your emotions, but to be in control of them. Consider the message you send with the emotion you show. Do suppress any urge to show your frustration toward kids who are trying to learn the skills, as well as any desire to express your anger on the field. Maintain your respect for the people involved in all situations. Your players need you to be steady and need to know what to expect from you.*

- **Not aware of nonverbal communication**—Some coaches watch what they say but not what they do. They express their frustration or anger nonverbally, and if someone confronts them about that expression, they likely will say, "What? I didn't say anything." *Remember that you're communicating every second,* *whether verbally or nonverbally. Keep your nonverbal communication in line with your verbal communication, and make sure that both are positive, instructive, and encouraging.*

■ **Buddy-buddy with the players**—It's good to be friendly with players, but it's inappropriate to try to be their friend. Coaches who do this show a lack of maturity as they try to impress their players with how cool they are. *Have fun with your players, but maintain the coach-player relationship. You're there to help them become better soccer players, not to become their pal.*

So, what *should* your communication style be?

You should provide the instruction your players need in a way that helps them improve their skills. To do this, you need good listening skills as well as good speaking skills, and you need to be encouraging and positive as you instruct and correct. Maintain respect for your players as you communicate with them. Be friendly and open with them, but don't try to become their friend. Create an enjoyable learning environment, maintain control over your emotions, and watch your nonverbal communication.

When you adopt this type of communication style, you're paving the way for your players to learn the game, improve their skills, and enjoy the season.

Be Receptive

A common mistake of new coaches is to assume that their sole role in communicating is to *talk*. Athletes are there to receive instruction, to be coached. Their focus should be on listening to you, on soaking in your instruction, on carrying out your commands.

There's plenty of truth in those statements, but they don't reflect the whole truth. Give your players room to speak, to ask questions, and to voice opinions or concerns. In doing so, you can get to know them better and be better tuned in to their needs. Thus, you will be more likely to pick up on issues and problems you need to deal with; see the following sidebar, "Dealing with Issues As They Arise."

Work at not only sending messages, but receiving them as well. As you talk to players, if you notice that their eyes are wandering or their bodies are turned partially away from you, they're sending you a message ("We're not really listening"). If their shoulders are slumped, their heads are down, or they're dragging their feet, they're sending one or more messages ("I'm tired"; "I'm

caution

Communication is a two-way street. If you make it one-way, athletes will eventually tune you out because you tuned them out when they attempted to talk to you.

discouraged"; "I'm bored"). If they're giving you a blank stare or have a dazed look, they're telling you they are tuning you out or are confused.

DEALING WITH ISSUES AS THEY ARISE

You might come across some discipline issues and other concerns you need to address as the season progresses. Here are some pointers on how to handle those issues:

- Let players know at the first practice how you expect them to behave, and let them know what the consequences of misbehavior will be. Write this down as well and give it to players or send it directly to their parents. This list needn't and shouldn't be long; it should be simple and clear and framed in a positive manner.

- Rather than just laying down the law, consider involving your players in making team rules. Do this at the first practice. When they take part in making the rules and setting the consequences for breaking them, they might be more apt to stick to the rules. Giving players this type of responsibility promotes their emotional and social growth.

- When a player misbehaves, follow through as you had said you would.

- Don't tolerate razzing of teammates, taunting of opposing players, or other poor sporting behavior. Put a stop to such behavior, and follow through on any prescribed penalties.

- When a player needs extra help at practice in learning a skill, try to provide it on the spot, ideally using an assistant coach or a parent who volunteers to help. If the help can't be provided during that practice, other options might be to provide further instruction immediately following the practice or immediately preceding the next practice, in a one-on-one situation, if possible.

- When a player needs medical attention, provide the appropriate care immediately. You'll learn about this care in Chapter 4, "Safety Principles."

Provide Helpful Feedback

Tyler has been having trouble distributing the ball as a goalkeeper. When he rolls the ball to a teammate, he tends to release it too high, causing it to bounce and slowing its progress. As a result, sometimes the opponents can sneak in and regain possession.

This, in fact, happens right before halftime in one game and the opponents get an easy goal because of Tyler's poor distribution. As Tyler approaches the sidelines for halftime, Coach Dixon approaches him and says, "Tyler, you need to do better than that."

Is Coach Dixon telling Tyler something he doesn't already know? Hardly. Is he helping Tyler improve his distribution technique? No. His feedback isn't helpful at all; if anything, it just adds to the pressure Tyler undoubtedly already feels.

Coach Dixon should focus on giving specific, practical feedback that will help Tyler improve his distribution technique—such as, "Tyler, remember to get low and release the ball smoothly at ground level, as if you were bowling." You'll learn about this type of feedback in Chapter 6, "Player Development." For now, know that such feedback is one of your duties in communicating with your players, and when it's given properly it can reap great dividends in terms of player improvement.

Be a Good Nonverbal Communicator

Studies have shown that up to 70% of communication is accomplished nonverbally. You just read about the importance of reading nonverbal cues—watching facial expressions and body language. You also have to pay attention to the nonverbal cues you send:

> "Way to go, Alex!" Coach Dintiman says, clapping his hands and smiling.
>
> "Way to go, Alex!" Coach Garner says, arms crossed tightly across his chest and a scowl on his face.

The same words were used, but Coach Garner sent a vastly different message from Coach Dintiman's.

Coaches constantly send nonverbal messages, both with and without words. Consider your facial expressions during practices and games. Sometimes it's appropriate to show that you're frustrated—for example, when kids are goofing off. But when kids are exerting themselves on the field and not executing well, keep your frustration in check. Consider what messages your expressions and body language are sending, and make sure those messages are what you *want* to be sending.

Be Consistent

Your players need consistency from you in three ways. They need consistency

- In the messages you send
- In how you treat them
- In your temperament and style

Consistent Messages

If you hear different messages from the same person on the same topic, what happens? You begin not to trust that person. The same happens if one week your players hear you say, "You guys need to tackle more! You're too passive. Be aggressive and go for the ball," only to hear you follow that the next week with, "You guys are trying to tackle too much. You're getting way out of position and being

caution
Remember, if your body language conflicts with your words, players will be just as confused as if you told them one thing one day and the opposite thing the next. Keep your body language in line with the verbal messages you send.

too aggressive." Confusing? You bet. If you do this often, the players will not know what to believe, no matter what you say. Be sure you send consistent messages.

Consistent Treatment

Be sure you treat all your players in a similar fashion. If Dana breaks a team rule one week and you discipline her accordingly and the next week Zach breaks the same rule, but you overlook it because he's one of your best players, what message does that send to your team? That it's okay to break the rules if you're good enough?

Likewise, if you spend more of your time with your average and good players, in hopes of turning them into good and great players, respectively, what does that say to the lesser-skilled players? That they don't matter because they can't dribble or shoot as well as their teammates?

All your players need your attention and guidance to improve. They need to adhere to the same team rules and be treated the same way if they break those rules. And they all need to know that they are equally valued by you, regardless of their playing ability.

Consistent Style

They also need to know what to expect from you. If you are patient and encouraging one practice and moody or volatile the next, the learning environment suffers (as do the players). We all have mood swings, and we're not robots. But do strive to be even-keeled and consistent in your approach from practice to practice, setting aside any personal issues that might affect your mood and your communication with your players on any given day.

Be Positive

Kids learn best in a positive environment. Give them sound instruction, consistent encouragement, and plenty of understanding. Note, however, that being positive doesn't mean letting kids run all over you, and it doesn't mean having a Pollyanna attitude where you falsely praise your midfielders for pursuing the ball when they should have gained possession of it. It means you instruct and guide your players as they learn and practice skills and give them the sincere encouragement and praise they need as they work to hone their abilities. You'll learn more about how to use praise in Chapter 6.

> **note**
>
> These 10 keys not only apply to how you communicate with your players, but also should guide your communication with parents, referees, other coaches, and administrators.

Communicating with Parents

While most communication happens between coaches and players, important communication takes place between coaches and parents, too. In this section, we'll consider the various times and ways you should communicate with parents and learn how to handle challenging situations and involve parents in positive ways throughout the season.

Preseason Meeting or Letter

You'll need to contact parents before the season begins. You can communicate the following information at a parents' meeting or through a letter. If you hold a parents' meeting, it's still helpful to give parents a handout that covers the items you talk about, so they can have written information to refer to later. In your preseason meeting or letter, consider including the following items:

- **Introduction**—Tell parents who you are, what your coaching background is (if you have one), and how you got involved coaching the team. Make this brief, but know that parents appreciate knowing a bit about who will be coaching their sons and daughters.

- **Your coaching philosophy**—Let parents know your approach to coaching, including your philosophy in terms of providing instruction, giving players equal playing time, and so on. Tell them, briefly, why this is your philosophy and how it benefits the kids.

- **The inherent risks**—Soccer has some inherent risks you need to make parents aware of. You should also let them know you have a plan in place to respond to injuries and find out from parents any medical conditions their children have, as well as how the parents can be contacted in case of an emergency. You'll learn more about this in Chapter 4.

- **Basic expectations**—State your expectations of players and parents, in a positive fashion, and let parents know what they and their children can expect of you as a coach.

- **The practice schedule**—Include the day, date, time, and place of the first practice, and note the rest of the practice schedule, if you know it at this time.

- **The game schedule**—If you know the game schedule, include that as well. If not, let parents know when they can expect to receive the schedule.

- **Other information**—If you have some special event planned or want to invite parents to volunteer to help in various ways, inform parents in your meeting or letter.

- **Your contact information**—Let parents know how and when they can contact you.

For a sample preseason letter, see Appendix A, "Sample Letter to Parents."

Preseason Call

Even with a preseason letter or meeting, it's wise to call parents of players before the first practice to remind them of the time and place of that practice. Otherwise, you'll likely have players who don't show up for the first practice.

During the Season

After the season is underway, you'll have numerous opportunities to communicate with parents: as kids are being dropped off or picked up at practice, after games, and on the phone or through email at other times of the week. Here are some pointers on doing so:

- If you have a few minutes immediately before or after practice, that's a good time to meet parents, get to know them a little bit, match faces with names, and enlist help if you need it. It's also a good time to let parents know what they can do to help their child. For example, you could suggest to Ramon's parents that if they had time, they could work with him at home on using the outer part of his foot to dribble, or you could let Tara's parents know she could use some practice receiving passes. Parents like to know what they can do to help their son or daughter.

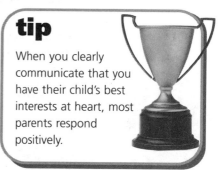

tip

When you clearly communicate that you have their child's best interests at heart, most parents respond positively.

- Ask parents to let you know when their child is not going to be at a game. Also let them know they can talk with you about any concerns they have about their child.

- Let parents know what type of communication is allowed during games. Whatever boundaries you set here, do so with the players in mind and what will help them focus on the game the most. Some coaches prefer not to have any direct parental intervention during a game, meaning shouting encouragement from the sidelines is fine, but going to the team area to talk to their child is not. Other coaches don't mind parents coming by and chatting briefly to the players; this is up to you. Just let parents know what your preferences are here, and ask that they respect them.

- Likewise, let parents know what's appropriate immediately after games. Many coaches like to spend 5 minutes or so talking to their players, reinforcing what went well and talking about what they still need to work on. At younger ages, post-game sometimes means snack time as well. Whatever your protocol, let parents know and let them know if and how they can be appropriately involved.

■ Rainouts or other types of cancellations call for communicating with parents, too. If a game or practice is cancelled or postponed, you can contact parents in whatever way you've set up: by yourself, with the aid of an assistant coach, or by phone tree. (A phone tree is a system that links all the families together. For example, on a team of 12 players, you could have 3 or 4 parents—the *branches*—call 3 or 4 families each, rather than you calling all 12 families. You should set up this tree beforehand.)

Whichever way you decide, though, make sure parents are contacted by phone when a practice or game is cancelled or postponed. Even if parents say email is a good way to contact them, chances are not all parents will check their email in time.

Be Understanding—and Set Boundaries

Most parents are there to cheer on their kids. Parents want to see their kids do their best, have fun, and succeed. It's thrilling for a parent to watch her child make a key pass that leads to a goal, make a great tackle, or score the winning goal. And it's painful for a parent to watch her son let a ball slip by him into the goal or see her daughter have the ball stolen from her in a crucial situation. It's likely that parents experience more emotional highs and lows watching their children play than do the players and coaches who are directly involved in the game.

You need to understand the experience from the parents' point of view and create an environment that allows parents to be positively involved throughout the season. Indeed, you should encourage such participation. (For suggestions on how to do this, see the following sidebar, "Involving Parents.")

At the same time, you need to set boundaries for parents and be prepared to handle situations that can detract from the players' experience. Some of those situations and boundaries are addressed in "Challenging Situations."

INVOLVING PARENTS

Some parents present challenges to coaches, but most want to support the team and its coach. Help parents know how they can be involved with your team in positive ways. Here are a few ideas:

■ **Encourage support**—Ask parents to be positive and vocal in their support of each player and to display good sporting behavior. Their main role at games is to cheer on their team.

■ **Ask for help**—If you don't have an assistant coach, ask if any parent would like to volunteer. Even if you do have an assistant, having parents volunteer to help at practice can be beneficial because you can break the players into smaller units and thus give them more touches on the ball. Also, you might want to set up parents on a snack schedule, with a different parent or set of parents responsible for providing a team snack at each game. Also, as previously mentioned, you also might set up a phone tree with parents so important information can be quickly passed on.

■ **Build camaraderie**—Social gatherings are nice ways to build camaraderie among parents and team family members. Consider having a midseason potluck or pizza party to help families get to know each other better, or plan other social events that foster open communication and deepened relationships. And parents are often more than willing to step to the fore and organize such events—so let them!

Challenging Situations

You might not have any challenging situations with parents. But it's best to be prepared for those challenges and know how to respond, just in case. Following are some of the challenges coaches can face and suggestions for how to handle them.

Parents Who Coach from the Sidelines

At some time during the season, you might experience the following:

> "You guys need to attack more! Defense, move up and help out on offense!" one parent yells during a game. "Switch to a 1-2-2!" another parent yells a little later. "Get the ball to Jason more!" a third parent adds.

It's one thing to encourage players from the sidelines; it's quite another to coach them from that vantage point. It's not a matter of whether the instruction is good; it's a matter of where that instruction is coming from. Coaching advice is your domain.

If you hear parents of your players coaching from the sidelines, remind your players to focus on what you say, not on what they hear elsewhere. Then, after the game, talk to the parents who were coaching from the sidelines. Tell them they need to focus their support on cheering on the team, not on telling them how to play. It's confusing and disconcerting for players to hear instruction from someone other than you, even if it's in line with what you've told them. And quite often that instruction flies in the face of what you've told them.

In any case, coaching from the sidelines is disruptive and inappropriate. Tell the offending parents this and request that they refrain from it in the future.

Parents Who Demand That You Coach Their Child Differently

There is also the possibility you will have parents who just don't think you are doing a good job with their child. Take some of the following sample comments:

> "My kid should be the goalie in our playoff game, not Derrick. If you want to win that game, you should be starting my kid as goalkeeper."

> "What's the deal with giving everyone all this playing time? My kid's the best player on the team, and he shouldn't be sitting out at all, unless it's a blowout."

"What are you doing playing my kid on defense? She's a much better forward than either of the guys you're playing there. She should be a forward, if you ask me."

Well, you *didn't* ask that parent, and you didn't ask the other parents for their "advice," either. But sometimes you get it, free of charge.

Don't get into a long conversation with parents on how you coach their child. You don't need to defend your right to make coaching decisions. Tell parents politely and firmly that while you appreciate their concerns, those are coaching decisions reserved for you and any assistant coaches you might have. Remind them that the decisions you make are in the best interest of all the players, including their own son or daughter. And leave it at that.

Parents Who Yell at Referees

If you've attended many youth soccer games, you've probably heard comments like the following:

"C'mon, ref! That was tripping!"

"Hey, ref! That kid is offside!"

"That's terrible! This guy calls it one way for one team and another way for the other team!"

Are parents justified in making derogatory or disparaging comments to or about referees? Absolutely not, even if the referee misses the call. Youth league referees are most often volunteers, unpaid and untrained. Yelling at the referee is poor sporting behavior, and it sends the wrong message to kids:

If I messed up, it was the referee's fault. If we lost, it was because of lousy refereeing.

It tells kids it's okay to disrespect the referee, it takes their focus off their own performance, and it implies that the game's outcome is far more important than it really is. It also usurps part of your role, which is to calmly discuss with referees certain calls (these debates should be rare; you'll learn more about them in "Communicating with Opponents and Referees," later in this chapter).

As noted earlier, let parents know up front what you expect of them, including their behavior at games. If they yell at the referees during games, talk with them after the game. Perhaps call them a little later in the evening, after they've had time to cool off. Tell them you appreciate their support but that you need them to stop berating the referees, even if they miss calls. Tell them why you feel this way (for the reasons stated in the previous paragraph), and ask that they refrain from doing so at future games.

Parents Who Yell at Their Own Kids

Parents who yell at their own kids—for missing a shot, for losing possession of the ball, for whatever reason—do a tremendous disservice to their children. The words of parents are extremely powerful, and they have the power to damage and destroy. Sadly, sports seem to be an arena in which some parents choose to harm their children's egos. Those damaging words reverberate in the youngster's ears long past the game and far from the field.

If a parent yells at his child during a game, counter the harmful words with your own words of encouragement and praise. Just make sure the praise is sincere because kids can see through false praise and such praise can undermine your own credibility and their ability to believe you in this or other situations.

If you believe the situation warrants it, talk to that parent during the game or send a nonverbal message to him to cut the negative talk. Before doing this, though, consider whether you can send your message without fanning the flames on the spot. You don't want an escalated confrontation; you want the parent to stop yelling at his kid.

If you don't communicate with the parent on the spot, do so after the game, one-on-one. Tell the parent that his son needs his support and encouragement. If he can't provide that support and encouragement, ask the parent to stop attending games.

Parents Who Yell at Other Kids

Many parents cheer on their own kids but loudly disparage other players, either on their own child's team or on the opposing team. Take the following examples:

> "Hey, this goalkeeper can't stop shots! We're going to score 10 goals today!"
>
> "Come on, you should've had that ball!"
>
> "Hey, nice shot, kid!" (A comment made with dripping sarcasm.)

Don't tolerate this any more than you would tolerate parents verbally abusing their own child. Intervene in the same way you would with a parent yelling at her own son or daughter.

note

What you're trying to do in all these situations is turn a win-lose situation into a win-win situation. You don't want to defeat parents; you want to win them over, so that you're on the same side, with the end result being that the players benefit.

Parents Who Abuse Their Children

Children can be abused physically, emotionally, and sexually. The signs of abuse are not always readily apparent, nor are they always easily separated from the scratches and bruises that come from normal childhood activity.

The point here is not to make you paranoid and suspect abuse when you see a player with a black eye, but to keep your own eyes open and watch for additional signs. Kids who are abused tend to

- Have a poor self-image
- Act out in practice or at games
- Be withdrawn, passive, or sad
- Lash out angrily at their peers
- Bully or intimidate weaker peers
- Have difficulty trusting others
- Be self-disparaging or self-destructive

Players who exhibit some or all of these signs might have been abused, or they might have experienced another child being abused. Complicating matters, these signs are also exhibited by kids who are undergoing various types of stress—for example, their parents' recent divorce.

If you do suspect that one of your players is being abused, it's your responsibility to contact the proper authorities—your local child protection services agency, police, your local hospital, or an emergency hotline. In many cases, you can do so anonymously. In any regard, if you have reason to believe abuse might be taking place, report it.

Communicating with League Administrators

Part of a league administrator's role is to set up and administer leagues. Administrators schedule games, set up league policies and rules, oversee the maintenance of the fields, dispense the necessary equipment, arrange for refereeing, and take care of many other responsibilities, all with the goal of providing a top-quality experience for the players.

A coach's interaction with league administrators generally falls into three categories:

- League information
- Coaches' meetings and clinics
- Questions and concerns

Let's look at each of these in the following sections.

League Information

The league should provide information on game schedules, practice field usage, equipment distribution, league policies and rules, and any upcoming coaches' meetings or clinics. Read the information you receive; make copies of the game schedules for parents; and talk with your administrator if you have any questions about the schedule, the policies, or any other information dispensed by the league.

Coaches' Meetings and Clinics

Most leagues hold a preseason coaches' meeting at which the administrator distributes the necessary information and updates coaches on new policies, modified rules, and other important matters.

Some leagues also conduct coaches' training. If your league offers such training, take advantage of it.

The point here is to consider ways to help you better prepare for your season. Coaching clinics and courses are one good way to do so.

> **tip**
>
> The American Sport Education Program (www.asep.com) offers effective training courses for youth coaches, including an online course in youth soccer. This is one of many good programs that can be found.

Questions and Concerns

Take any overarching questions or concerns—about league policies or rules, practice field availability, scheduling, and so on—to your league administrator. In addition, if you have an ongoing problem with a parent and are unable to resolve it with that parent, consider talking with your league administrator. By all means, do so if the problem affects the enjoyment of the game for other fans, the parent poses some sort of physical threat to anyone, or the parent is verbally abusive at games and refuses to stop or leave when she becomes abusive.

Communicating with Opponents and Referees

Three key words here: *respect*, *dignity*, *restraint*.

Besides being your players' coach, you are also their role model, whether you like it or not. And how you communicate with opposing coaches, players, and referees speaks volumes about what kind of role model you are.

If you have a question for a referee, ask it at the proper time and without showing up the referee or unnecessarily slowing the game. Treat the referees, and the opposing coaches, with the same respect you'd like to be shown.

At the ends of games, line up your players and lead them as you shake hands with the other

> **note**
>
> You can teach your kids all the requisite skills, but if you don't teach them how to play the game—all-out, having fun, and showing respect for the referees and opponents—you haven't taught them enough.

team. Instruct your players to be respectful as they shake or slap hands. Also thank the referees for volunteering their time.

THE ABSOLUTE MINIMUM

This chapter was all about what, when, and how to communicate with your players, parents, league administrators, opposing coaches and players, and referees. Key points included

- Use the 10 keys to being a good communicator. Those keys are 1) Know your message; 2) Make sure you are understood; 3) Deliver your message in the proper context; 4) Use appropriate emotions and tones; 5) Adopt a healthy communication style; 6) Be receptive; 7) Provide helpful feedback; 8) Be a good nonverbal communicator; 9) Be consistent; and 10) Be positive.

- Contact parents before the season begins, sharing information about your coaching philosophy and practice and game schedules and paving the way for healthy communication throughout the season.

- Let parents know what you expect of them, in terms of positive team support, and what they can expect of you.

- Suggest ways parents can be actively involved in supporting and helping the team.

- Work through the challenging situations parents sometimes present. Keep your players' best interests in mind as you work for win-win situations.

- If you have reason to believe a player has been abused, report it to local authorities.

- Give the referees and opponents the same respect you would like to be shown. Be a model of good sporting behavior for your players.

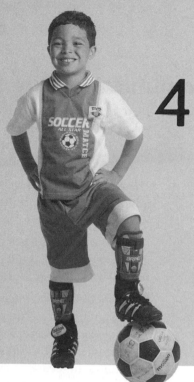

4

Safety Principles

Soccer isn't a contact sport. But it is a sport that involves a lot of running, and collisions do happen. Add in balls that are kicked, less-than-perfect field conditions, and young bodies that aren't always in complete control of themselves, and it's no wonder injuries occur in soccer.

Sometimes these injuries are preventable, and sometimes they aren't. This chapter focuses on how to create a safe environment for your players, provide the supervision they need, and do all you can to prevent injuries. You'll also learn how to respond to the injuries that do happen. Hopefully you won't have an emergency to respond to, but if you do, you need to know what action to take, so you'll learn about that as well. Finally, we'll consider safety precautions related to severe weather.

Communicating the Inherent Risk

Three players converge on a ball, colliding as they go for it. A hard shot zings off a young goalkeeper's face before he can get his hands up. A youngster, trying to make a cut on the field, twists his ankle. Another player gets unintentionally kicked as she goes for the ball.

These are just some of the ways players get injured in soccer. Most of the injuries are minor—scrapes, cuts, bruises, muscle cramps and spasms, and muscle strains. Major injuries are rare, but they can occur.

Like all sports, soccer has its inherent risks. It's your duty to communicate these risks to parents. As mentioned in Chapter 3, "Communication Keys," you should do this before the season starts, either in a letter or in a parent meeting.

What should you say? Tell the parents about the types of injuries that can occur. Assure them that you will do everything in your power to prevent injuries, but that you can't prevent all injuries, and parents and players should understand the risks going in.

Ask parents to do their part, meaning equipping their children with adequate footwear (rubber cleats are preferable to provide traction) and shin guards. Let parents know you will do your part in providing adequate supervision at practices and games.

Many leagues have consent forms parents must fill out. In doing so, parents acknowledge that they understand the risks involved and do not hold the coach or the league liable for injuries that occur while players are participating in the program.

caution

Consent forms do not protect you from all liability issues. If you do not provide adequate supervision or respond appropriately to an injured player, you can still be held liable. However, by being able to prove that you provided proper supervision and instruction, you are less likely to be held accountable for a player's injury.

Being Prepared

There are several actions you can take to prepare for injuries and emergency situations. Three of those actions include

- Having CPR/first aid training
- Being prepared to respond to kids with chronic health conditions
- Having a well-stocked first aid kit on hand

Beyond these, you should also have a plan for responding to both minor injuries and major injuries. You'll learn more about those plans a little later in this chapter. For now, let's take a look at the three items just mentioned.

CPR/First Aid Training

CPR and first aid training is often offered through local hospitals and medical clinics, as well as through national organizations such as the American Red Cross. Sports leagues often sponsor or arrange for the training, which covers the basics of providing cardiopulmonary resuscitation and first aid for a variety of injuries.

If you have the opportunity to be trained in CPR/first aid, take it. Understanding the proper response and practicing the correct techniques involved go much further than reading about the topic.

If you don't have the opportunity to be trained, study this chapter carefully and supplement your learning with additional resources as you see fit.

Chronic Health Condition Awareness

Dontrelle, after playing midfielder for about 5 minutes, begins to wheeze hard as play is about to resume with a throw-in. He can't seem to catch his breath. His wheezing is beyond the normal out-of-breath, out-of-shape gasping for air. He is truly having trouble getting enough air into his lungs. What do you do?

Hannah is stung by a bee and her eyes begin to itch and swell. She develops hives and begins wheezing. How do you respond?

Tyler begins sweating and trembling. He is turning pale. You know he is diabetic. What action do you take?

Dontrelle has asthma; Hannah is allergic to bee stings; and Tyler, as mentioned, suffers from diabetes. These are examples of chronic conditions some of your players might have and that you might have to deal with as your season progresses. With chronic health conditions, it's vital that you

- Are aware that the child has the condition.
- Know the signs the child will exhibit when the condition is bothering him or her.
- Know how to respond to the symptoms.

Before the first practice, have parents fill out a medical emergency form (see Appendix B, "Medical Emergency Form"). On this form they can note which type of allergy or condition their child has, which symptoms to watch for, what to do in case of an attack or episode, and at what phone numbers they can be reached.

If parents note an allergy or condition but are sparse with their information on what signs to look for, ask them directly what you should watch for. You can also find this information easily on the Internet or through resources in your library.

Just as important as knowing what to look for is knowing how to respond. The child's parents are the first and most important resource here; they will know what treatment is called for. Some situations will call for you to seek immediate emergency help. Know what these situations are and carry the appropriate medical emergency numbers—and a cell phone, if possible—with you at practices and games. If you don't have a cell phone, carry change with you for a pay phone.

First Aid Kit

Stock a first aid kit and take it with you to practices and games. Some stores sell complete kits; you can buy an already-assembled kit or put one together on your own. Either way, here are the essentials you should have on hand:

- Phone numbers of parents, players' doctors, emergency medical personnel, and police
- Change for a pay phone
- Antiseptic wipes
- Antibacterial soap
- First aid cream
- Instant cold pack
- Gauze rolls
- Triangular bandages
- 2" elastic bandage
- Bandages, sheer and flexible, of various sizes
- Nonstick pads of assorted sizes
- Hypoallergenic first aid tape
- Oval eye pads
- Acetaminophen
- Scissors
- Tweezers
- Insect sting kit
- Disposable gloves
- First aid guide
- Contents card

tip

Use the contents card to remind you of what you *should* have and what you *do* have, so you know when to restock. Use the first aid guide to help you remember how to care for minor injuries (it's easier than carrying this book with you to practice).

Providing Proper Supervision

In the rush to provide superior coaching and teaching, to shape their youngsters into the best possible soccer players over the course of a season, many coaches overlook an even more important duty: to provide proper supervision at practices and games.

Parents are entrusting their children to you; your most important duty is to make sure their kids are cared for and supervised in a safe environment.

To provide the supervision your players need, be sure you

- Plan your practices.
- Inspect the field and equipment.
- Provide proper instruction.
- Supervise each activity.

Plan Your Practices

In Chapter 5, "Practice Plans," you'll learn how to plan your season and individual practices. Planning prepares you to instruct and coach more effectively. When you're organized and know what you want to teach, and how you want to teach it, you're more likely to stay on task and maintain control. In turn, your players are more likely to stay focused, taking their cues from you, and less likely to have down time to fool around while you're figuring out what to do next.

You'll learn to plan your practices using a logical progression of skills, based on your players' level of development and physical condition.

Keep these season and practice plans; they can be important if an injury were to occur and your judgment in terms of planning were questioned. Also fill out and keep any injury reports (see Appendix C, "Injury Report") for your records.

Inspect the Field and Equipment

Check your practice and game fields before playing on them. Look for holes, broken glass, rocks, and other items—either part of the natural terrain or manmade—that pose a threat to your players. If there are hazards on the field that you can't remove or fix, do whatever you can to reduce the risks they present and warn your players about them. Then report those hazards to your league administrator.

Inspect the equipment your players use, as well. Make sure each player is wearing properly fitted shin guards.

Provide Proper Instruction

If your players don't know how to spread out their attack, they're more likely to clot up around the ball, which leads to greater chance of injury. Likewise, if your players don't know how to properly mark and tackle, they are more likely to get hurt when they attempt to do so. And if your goalkeepers don't know the proper techniques for defending the goal, they increase their chances of being injured.

That's why it's important that you teach your players the proper technique for all the skills they need to perform. It not only increases their chances of playing well, but also decreases their chances of being injured.

Supervise Each Activity

Planning the practice, knowing what you want your players to be doing from minute to minute, isn't enough. You need to closely supervise the players as they participate in each activity. Accidents and injuries are more likely to happen when activities are not supervised.

That means don't get kids started in an activity and then watch them out of the corner of your eye while you make a call on your cell phone. It also means not temporarily leaving the practice field, leaving the players in the charge of your teenage son. It means staying focused on the activity, being there to provide feedback on players' performances, and—most importantly from a legal standpoint—ensuring that the activity is conducted safely and that all players are under your direct supervision.

For additional ways to make practices safe, see the following sidebar, "Safety Tips."

SAFETY TIPS

Here are three more ways to provide for your players' safety:

- **Remember that your players are kids, not miniature adults**—Their bodies can't take the physical stress that adult bodies can. Don't encourage kids to play through pain, and don't expect them to do what you can do.

- **Stretch and warm up properly for practices and games**—Lead your players through a warm-up routine that includes a few minutes of easy running followed by stretching.

- **Make clear rules pertaining to when and where players can kick balls, and enforce the rules**—Otherwise, players will be kicking balls that are on the sideline at practice when they shouldn't be, and when other players aren't looking for the ball.

Responding to Minor Injuries

The focus so far has been on doing all you can to prevent injuries from occurring. Still, they will occur, and you need to know how to respond to them.

Most of the injuries in youth soccer are minor: cuts and scrapes, bruises, sprains, and strains. Here's how you should respond in each situation.

Cuts and Scrapes

Remember the disposable gloves in your first aid kit? Here's where you use them: as a barrier between you and a player's blood. While wearing the gloves, stop the bleeding by pressing directly on the cut with a gauze bandage. If the cut is deep enough that blood soaks the bandage, keep that bandage in place and apply another one.

When the bleeding has stopped, remove the gauze bandage and cleanse the wound with an antiseptic wipe. Apply some first aid cream. Then place a clean bandage over the wound.

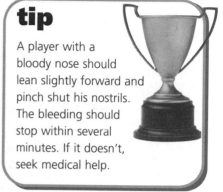

tip

A player with a bloody nose should lean slightly forward and pinch shut his nostrils. The bleeding should stop within several minutes. If it doesn't, seek medical help.

Bruises

Things sometimes go bump in the night. More often, they go bump at midfield, or near the goal, or in the corner as three players chase down an errant pass. Wherever the bump takes place, a bruise often results. Many bruises don't need any special treatment, but if the area is swollen and tender, treat it through the PRICE method:

- **P = Protect**—Keep the athlete from further harm as you tend to the injury.
- **R = Rest**—This hastens the healing process.
- **I = Ice**—This reduces inflammation in the injured area, which aids in the healing process; it also reduces the pain.
- **C = Compress**—When you compress the injured area with a tightly secured ice bag (use an elastic bandage to do this), you ensure that the ice can do its job.
- **E = Elevate**—When you raise the injured area above the heart level, this minimizes the amount of blood that pools in the area. The more blood that pools in the area, the longer the injury will take to heal.

tip

Apply ice for about 15 minutes every 3 hours or so during the day. When the swelling decreases, the player can begin gentle range-of-motion exercises for the affected joint.

Sprains and Strains

A *sprain* happens when ligaments or tendons are stretched too far from their normal position. Typically, a sprain occurs in the ankle, knee, or wrist. A sprain generally causes pain, swelling, and bruising of the affected joint.

A *strain* occurs when a muscle is stretched too far. In soccer, the most common strains are to hamstrings, the muscles in the backs of the thighs. A strained hamstring generally relates to a single, specific incident—for example, sprinting to reach a ball, or lunging to stop a shot.

> **note**
>
> Overuse injuries result from the stress placed on bodies by repetitive training. Such injuries can include stress fractures, strains, sprains, tendonitis, bursitis, and shin splints.

Treat sprains and strains with the PRICE method. The player should fully recover and gradually work back to full speed.

Remember to use the injury report to keep a record of all injuries, including minor ones.

RETURNING AFTER AN INJURY

Most players want to return from an injury as soon as possible. But if they return too quickly, they can aggravate the injury and end up missing more action than necessary.

Here are some guidelines for when injured players can return to action:

- They should return when they have been cleared to do so by their parents and, if appropriate, by their doctor.
- They should not practice or play if they still feel pain in the injured area during rest.
- They should use simple exercises to gently work the injured area once they have no pain at rest.
- If they feel pain as they resume exercising, they should stop.
- They should return gradually to full intensity, listening to their bodies and increasing intensity only when they can do so without pain.

Responding to Emergency Situations

You need to be prepared to respond to emergency situations such as broken bones and head, neck, and back injuries. An emergency situation can also crop up with a chronic health condition. Your role here is not to treat the player, but to facilitate that treatment while protecting the player from further harm.

To do so, you need to have an emergency plan in place. Here are the essentials of such a plan:

1. Evaluate the player and use your CPR/first aid training as appropriate. However, do *not* move, or allow the movement of, a player who has suffered a neck or back injury, a dislocated joint, or a broken bone.

2. Contact medical personnel, reassure the child, keep others away from him, and remain with the child until medical help arrives. Assign an assistant coach or a parent to call medical personnel, if possible. It's ideal that you stay with the player to keep him calm.

3. If the child is taken to the hospital and his parents are not available to go with him, appoint an assistant coach or a parent to accompany the child. Ideally, this person will be someone the player knows and can take comfort from.

tip

Always carry these phone numbers with you at practices and games: players' parents (home, office, and mobile phones), players' physicians, hospital, police, and rescue unit. Also be sure you have players' emergency information on hand. You'll gain this information through the form found in Appendix B.

Heatstroke

In heatstroke, a person's body temperature climbs dangerously high as heat is generated more quickly than the body can handle it. As the body's thermoregulatory mechanisms fail, heatstroke can occur. In the late stages of heatstroke, the person loses his ability to sweat, but this isn't the case earlier on.

Signs of heatstroke include

- Fatigue and weakness
- Nausea and vomiting
- Headache
- Dizziness
- Muscle cramps
- Irritability

A person suffering from heatstroke has hot, flushed skin. She likely also has a rapid pulse, shallow breathing and constricted pupils. The person might exhibit strange behavior and confusion.

What should you do if a player exhibits some of these signs? Get the player into shade, have her sit or lie down, remove any excess clothing or equipment, and cool her body with wet towels or by pouring cold water over her. Have someone call medical personnel immediately. Have the player drink cool water. Another way to cool the body is to place ice packs on the armpits, neck, and back and between the legs.

Under no circumstances should you allow an athlete who has suffered heatstroke to return to action until she has been examined by a doctor and cleared to play.

Heat Exhaustion

Heat exhaustion happens when a person becomes dehydrated. This person usually is sweating profusely and has pale, clammy skin; a rapid and weak pulse; dilated pupils; and a loss of coordination.

The signs of heat exhaustion are the same as for heatstroke. The treatment is also the same, with the exception that you might not need to send for medical personnel. Send for medical personnel if the player's condition doesn't improve or if it worsens. Again, don't let the player resume practicing or playing without the consent of her physician.

> **caution**
>
> About 200 people in the United States die each year due to heat-related illnesses. The chance of death increases when treatment is delayed for more than 2 hours. Don't delay in treating your players for heat-related illnesses and in seeking medical intervention when necessary.

Respecting the Weather

The weather can present significant threats to the well-being of players and coaches. In this section, you'll learn about guidelines for three weather-related situations: heat, lightning, and severe weather.

Heat Guidelines

Heatstroke and heat exhaustion most commonly occur in hot, humid weather. To help prevent heat illnesses, use caution in hot climates. Here are some guidelines for exercising in the heat:

- Realize it takes a week or two for the body to adapt to a hot environment. That means if you've had a cool spring and suddenly a heat wave strikes, the heat will affect your players more in that first week or two.
- When it's hot, train before 10 a.m. or after 4 p.m. if possible.
- Make sure your players wear loose-fitting, light-colored clothing because it's coolest and allows more sweat to evaporate.

- Encourage your players to drink water before they come to practice, and have water on hand at practice. You might suggest that your players bring their own water bottles. They should drink about 4–6 ounces of water every 20 minutes in hot or humid conditions. Tell them to drink plenty of water after practice as well.

- On hot or humid days, take a 5- to 10-minute water break in the middle of practice. Get in the shade while you do so.

Lightning Guidelines

Your league might have lightning guidelines in place; if so, follow those. If not, use the *flash-to-bang method* to determine your response. After you see a flash of lightning, begin counting seconds. Stop counting when you hear thunder. For every 5 seconds you count, the lightning is 1 mile away. So, if you count 10 seconds, the lightning is 2 miles away; if you count 15 seconds, the lightning is 3 miles away; and so on.

You should take immediate defensive action when lightning is indicated within 6–8 miles (30–40 "flash-to-bang" seconds). Why? Because the next bolt of lightning can strike 6–8 miles away from the previous strike. Don't be fooled into thinking it's far away; *it isn't*.

When lightning is within 6–8 miles, do the following:

- Stop playing or practicing. Seek shelter immediately inside a safe structure (one with four walls). The safest shelters have electrical and telephone wiring as well as plumbing because these aid in grounding the structure.

- If you cannot find such a shelter, a fully enclosed vehicle with a metal roof is your next best choice. The windows should be completely closed. It is important that you not touch any part of the metal framework of the vehicle while inside it as the storm is occurring.

- Avoid high points in open fields. Don't stand under or near trees, flagpoles, or light poles.

If you feel your hair stand on end, feel your skin tingle, or hear crackling noises, assume the lightning safety position. Crouch on the ground with your weight on the balls of your feet. Keep your feet together, lower your head, and cover your ears. Do *not* lie flat on the ground.

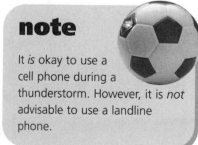

note

It *is* okay to use a cell phone during a thunderstorm. However, it is *not* advisable to use a landline phone.

Severe Weather Guidelines

Don't hold practice if there is a tornado or severe weather watch or warning for your area. If a tornado or severe storm watch or warning occurs after you have begun practice or a game, seek immediate shelter in the nearest building.

If no buildings are nearby, the next best thing is to head for the lowest ground, preferably in a ditch or ravine. If a bridge or highway overpass is nearby, it can offer shelter as well. Get as close as you can to the top and hold tightly to the supports.

Unlike the protection they can offer to those trying to avoid lightning, cars are one of the worst places you can be with a tornado approaching.

THE ABSOLUTE MINIMUM

This chapter is intended to prepare you to provide for the safety of your players. Among the main points are these:

- Let parents know of the inherent risks of playing soccer before the season begins.

- There are many ways you can prepare yourself to provide for safety. Among them are being trained in CPR/first aid, being aware of any chronic health conditions of your players, knowing how to respond if a player's health condition flares up, and having a well-stocked first aid kit on hand at all practices and games.

- One of your most important duties is to provide proper supervision at practices and games. This comes through planning your practices, inspecting the field and equipment, providing proper instruction, and closely supervising each activity.

- Know how to respond to minor injuries, including cuts and scrapes, bruises, and sprains and strains.

- Have an emergency plan in place, have all the important phone numbers you need in case of an emergency, and enact the plan when a major injury happens.

- Respect the weather. Know the guidelines for exercising in the heat and be aware of the symptoms of heat illness and how you should respond to it. Also know the guidelines for taking cover when lightning or severe weather is in the area.

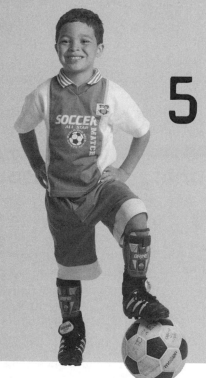

IN THIS CHAPTER

- Planning your season
- Planning practices
- Conducting your first practice
- 12 keys to conducting effective practices

5

PRACTICE PLANS

Generally, the people who volunteer their time—such as for coaching—are already busy people. Now they add one more thing to their plate. And then, in the few quiet moments of their day (usually lasting no more than 30 seconds), they wonder how they are going to find the time to fulfill their latest volunteer obligations.

Many inexperienced coaches, pressed for time and unaware of the harm they are doing, go into and through the season winging it from practice to practice. Their argument is simple: They don't have the time to prepare.

You don't need to spend massive amounts of time in preparation for your season and practices. But spending some preparation time will greatly aid your coaching efforts.

So, use this chapter to help you prepare for your season and practices. You will be glad you did—and your players will be, too. Your practices will run more smoothly, with less down time. Your players will learn all they need to learn, and in a logical order. And you will get the most out of your limited time with your players.

Planning Your Season

If you plan from practice to practice without keeping the big picture in mind, you risk overlooking some tactics or skills you should be teaching; you also risk presenting the skills you do teach in less than an ideal order. For example, it's no good teaching your players how to make first-touch passes if they can't adequately receive and control a pass on the second or third touch yet. They need to hone their basic passing and receiving skills before they attempt first-touch passes. Likewise, if your players haven't gotten the hang of basic marking, it's not the right time to teach them to tackle.

When you develop a season plan, then, consider what you should teach throughout the season and when you should teach it.

These three elements will help you construct a plan for your season:

- Purpose
- Tactics and skills
- Rules

Purpose

You should have an overall purpose for every practice, and, when considered in context of the entire season, there should be a logical flow to the purpose of each practice. For example, the purposes in the early-season practices should be to introduce and teach the basic skills. As the season progresses, the purposes should become to refine the basic skills and learn the tactics related to those skills (and to learn more complex skills, if appropriate for the age you're coaching).

Having a purpose gives the practice an informed drive and energy. You and your players are there for a particular reason that day, and your time is spent in trying to accomplish the goals for that practice.

Tactics and Skills

Based on the purpose of the practice, you will focus on teaching a particular skill or tactic. That doesn't mean your players don't practice other tactics or skills during that practice, but that the main emphasis is on learning or refining a particular skill or tactic.

When you lay out, in a season plan, all the skills and tactics you plan to teach, it helps to ensure that you don't overlook something important and that your teaching has a logical flow.

Rules

Many coaches overlook teaching rules to their players. Don't assume your players know the rules. Plan to take some time to teach the basic rules; your players need to know these as much as they need to develop their skills. When you make plans to teach the basic rules, you're much more likely to take the time to do so.

Adjusting Your Season Plan

If you are coaching 6- and 7-year-olds, your season plan will be simpler than if you were coaching 9- and 10-year-olds. As kids gain in size, experience, and physical abilities, they are able to learn more advanced skills and tactics. In general, keep your plans simple and adjust them as you need to based on your players' abilities.

> **tip**
>
> Teach rules within the context of playing. Set up an offside situation, briefly explain and demonstrate the rule, and then practice it (instructing the player in the offside position to move toward the sideline, away from the play, so she won't be called for being offside). Players learn rules much better in an action context, as opposed to you simply telling them the rules.

If they've demonstrated they have picked up the basics more quickly than you thought they would, step up your plans a bit. For example, if your 11- and 12-year-olds have demonstrated that they can pretty consistently penetrate the defense as they attack, you might teach them to further orchestrate their attack by using a target player to feed the shooter.

On the other hand, if you have planned to introduce the use of a target player by mid-season and your players still have difficulty in penetrating the defense, keep your focus on developing more fundamental attack skills before moving on to the target player idea. It might be that you never do move on to that concept during that season.

The main point is to adjust your plan to what the players need.

Sample Season Plan

Table 5.1 contains a sample 8-week season plan for a 9- and 10-year-old team that meets once a week. This model is *not* meant to be the one-and-only way to plan your season; it is one example, intended to give you a start. Use it as a guide when you construct your own season plan. Appendix D, "Season Plan," has a blank season plan you can use.

Create your season plan before the season begins. Construct a plan that reflects however many times you will practice throughout the season. Plan your season the way you believe will work best for your players, so long as you cover the basics first and move at a pace that is good for them, adjusting as need be.

note

Although you list one main purpose for each practice, you can and should work on multiple skills in a single practice.

TABLE 5.1   8-week Practice Plan

Week	Purpose	Tactics/Skills	Rules
1	Learning basic offensive skills	Dribbling	Learning positions
		Passing	Handball
		Receiving	Kickoff
2	Learning basic defensive skills	Marking	Fouls (kicking, striking)
		Goalkeeping	Direct free kick
			Goalkeeper rules
3	Learning a basic defensive skill	Tackling	Fouls (tripping, holding, pushing, and charging into an opponent)
			Indirect free kick
4	Learning basic offensive skills	Shooting	Offside
		Heading	Penalty kick
5	Learning offensive tactics	Spreading the attack	Corner kick
		Providing support	Throw-in
		Give-and-go	
		Corner kicks and throw-ins	
6	Learning defensive tactics	Channeling the opponent to the weaker side	Goal kick
		Defending corner kicks and throw-ins	
7	Reviewing and refining	Practicing the skills and tactics needed most	
8	Reviewing and refining	Practicing the skills and tactics needed most	

Planning Practices

After you have your season plan in place, you can begin to construct your practice plans. Create your practice plans one at a time—that is, don't create your entire season's worth of practice plans at once because you might find you need to adjust them based on what your players need most to focus on.

This section covers the essential structure of your practices; in the upcoming section "12 Keys to Conducting Effective Practices," we delve into the methods that will help you run successful practices within the structure presented here.

The Best Option: Simultaneous Stations

Soccer coaches have two basic options in structuring their practices. One option is to have all the players together, receiving instruction and then practicing the skills and tactics in one large group. Advantages to this option are that all the players receive the exact same instruction and the coach can easily view the action and provide feedback because only one station is being used. The downfall is that practice time isn't being maximized; players are standing around, waiting for their turn to pass or shoot or mark. With only one ball in play and about 15 players, that's an inefficient way to practice. Players learn and develop their skills less and have more time to goof off.

The better option is to give instruction to the entire team and then run simultaneous stations. After a team warm-up, split the team into three groups and set up three stations. After every 15 minutes, instruct each group to rotate to a new station. By the end of practice, each group will have had 15 minutes at each of the three stations. (With a 5- to 10-minute warm-up and a 5-minute wrap-up, that makes for a 60-minute practice.) In this way, players are active and engaged, they receive more chances to improve their skills, and they're having more fun.

Which stations you set up depend on what you are focusing on. Figures 5.1 and 5.2 show two examples of setting up three-station fields.

In Figure 5.1, group 1 begins with passing and receiving practice; group 2 begins with marking practice; and group 3 practices shooting and goalkeeping. In Figure 5.2, group 1 begins with ball control practice; group 2 begins with heading practice; and group 3 begins with tackling practice. Again, in each instance, the groups rotate after 15 minutes.

Simultaneous situations can provide the best learning experiences for players and make practices more active and fun, but they can also present challenges. You need to be aware of those challenges and know how to overcome them. There are two primary challenges: ensuring player safety and maintaining the quality of instruction and feedback provided to players.

FIGURE 5.1
Plan one for
three-station
practices.

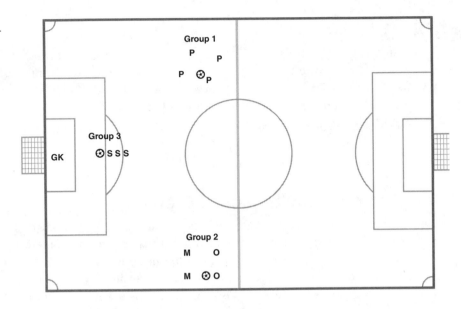

GK – goalkeeper   P – passer
S – shooter   M – marker
⊛ – ball   O – offense

FIGURE 5.2
Plan two for
three-station
practices.

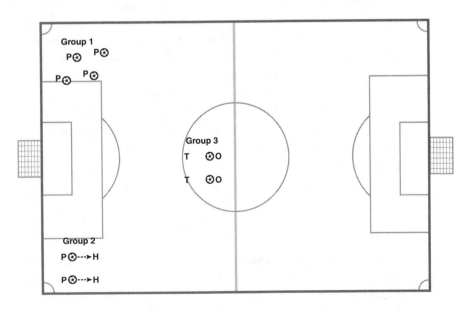

⊛ – ball   H – header   T – tackler
P – player   O – offense

Player Safety

Set up your stations in a way that allows the players at each station to not be infringed upon by play from another station. As for supervision, the ideal is to have one adult per station. So, to run three simultaneous stations, you ideally would use three adults.

Do you *need* three adults to safely supervise three stations? No. Some experienced coaches have safely run simultaneous stations by themselves. In this case, you would set up each station, get players going in each, and move from station to station, observing and providing feedback.

In a better scenario, you will have an assistant coach. (If an assistant hasn't been assigned to you, ask the parents of your players if one or more would like to assist you. Generally, at least one parent will offer to help.) The setup time for the stations is quicker with an assistant available, and one coach can watch two stations while the other watches the third.

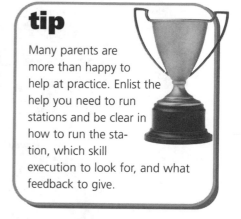

tip

Many parents are more than happy to help at practice. Enlist the help you need to run stations and be clear in how to run the station, which skill execution to look for, and what feedback to give.

In the best scenario, you will have an assistant coach and some parent volunteers who can aid in watching and running stations. In this way, you could have an adult at each station providing feedback.

If you have an assistant coach and no other volunteers, you should still be able to run simultaneous stations. The drawback is you can't provide all the feedback you'd like because you can't be two places at once. You move from station to station, and you can be at one station and observe some of the action from another station, or you can stand between two stations and observe much of the action from both, but it's not the same as being at one station, focused only on the players and the action there.

But it's still worth it because the players get more skill practice this way. You just have to make sure you provide the instruction and feedback they need.

Coaching Instruction and Feedback

Of course, the primary purpose of the simultaneous stations is to give players more practice at skill execution. But if Damon is continually kicking the ball too far from himself as he dribbles, is he going to improve his dribbling skills? Not likely.

Players need feedback on their skill execution. They need to know what's right, what's wrong, and how to fix what's wrong. It's that feedback that helps them learn and improve.

When you have a coach or parent volunteer at each station, you are in the best situation for providing that feedback. Realize, however, that many parents might not know precisely what to look for or what feedback to provide; tell any volunteer exactly what to look for and what type of feedback to give. Give volunteers the easier stations to run, in terms of providing feedback.

Sample Practice Plan

In Appendix E, "Practice Plan," you'll find a blank practice plan you can photocopy and use. See Figure 5.3 for a sample 60-minute practice plan.

FIGURE 5.3

A 60-minute practice plan.

Sample Practice Plan

Date April 15   **Place** Coles Field   **Time** 5:30 p.m.

Equipment Balls, cones, pinnies

Purpose Learning passing, receiving, dribbling

Activity	Description	Time	Comments
1. Warm-up	Run, stretch	5 min	Focus them on practice purpose
2. Passing and Receiving	*Instruction:* Passing and receiving techniques	5 min	Split into groups of three. *Passing:* Short passes with inside of foot. Longer passes with shoelace area. *Receiving:* Cushion ball. Keep it close to you.
	Game: Triangle Passing	10 min	Pairs passing and receiving within a triangle marked with cones.
3. Dribbling	*Instruction:* Dribbling technique	5 min	Both sides of feet. Keep ball close. Look up! Keep in control.
	Game: Follow the Leader	10 min	Pair up. Dribbler follows the leader, who jogs ahead of dribbler.
4. Water break		5 min	
5. Scrimmage	6v6	15 min	1 point for successful passes, 2 points for goals
6. Cool-down		5 min	Instructional reminders. Next practice reminder.

Notes

Need more work on making strong, accurate passes and on controlling passes. Also on keeping ball close when dribbling and seeing the field as you dribble.

Here are a few things to note about the sample plan:

- Instruction time is allotted for each of the stations. You won't always need to allot time for instruction, though. If you have already instructed your players on the skill or tactic, you can start the station with a drill or game.

- Most of the time at a station should be spent in games or drills. You'll learn more about setting up games and drills in "12 Keys to Conducting Effective Practices."

- The Comments section is meant for you to write coaching tips and technique reminders you want to focus on in that station.

- The Notes section is for things you observe as the players perform at each station. Use this section to jot down observations you want to bring up at the end of practice or techniques you want to work on at the next practice, and use it to keep a log or journal of each player's progress.

Conducting Your First Practice

Your first practice is different from all the other practices in a few respects. First, you're probably meeting the majority of your players for the first time, so introductions are in order. Second, you want to create, at the outset, the proper environment, one that balances fun with learning. Your players need to understand that you're there to help them learn and improve their skills. They also need to know what to expect from you and what you expect from them.

You can accomplish this in relatively short order—probably taking 5–10 minutes. From there, you can conduct your practice as normal.

Structure your first practice like this:

1. **Introduction (5–10 minutes)**—Coach and player introductions (kids enjoy a fun icebreaker game here). Goals for the season. Your expectations of players and what they can expect of you. The practice structure. Team rules and safety issues. See the following sidebar, "Setting the Tone," for more detail on this first-practice introduction.

2. **Warm-up (5–10 minutes)**—Light running and stretching.

3. **Station 1 (10–15 minutes)**—Dribbling instruction and practice.

4. **Station 2 (10–15 minutes)**—Passing and receiving instruction and practice.

5. **Station 3 (10–15 minutes)**—Shooting and goalkeeping practice.

6. **Wrap-up (5 minutes)**—Reinforce what most needs to be reinforced, based on activities. Remind players of the next practice or game.

SETTING THE TONE

To get off on the right foot, you need to communicate certain messages in the first practice and set the tone for a good learning environment. Some things to consider covering in that first practice are

- **Goals for the season**—Briefly tell players your goals for the season, which should be centered on helping them improve their skills, increase their understanding of the game, and have fun.

- **Your expectations**—Let them know that you expect them to show up on time for practice, to pay attention to your instruction and feedback, to obey any rules you set up (mainly concerned with safety), to give full effort, to respect others, to ask questions if they don't understand something, to ask for help when they need it, and to tell you if they are hurt.

- **What players can expect**—Also let players know what to expect from you: that you're there to provide instruction, feedback, and encouragement and to help each player improve his or her skills.

- **Practice structure**—Briefly let players see the big picture of how a typical practice will go.

- **Team rules/safety issues**—Inform players of your rules regarding kicking balls. Also talk about sideline protocol (or you might address this prior to the first game). Don't go overboard on rules, but do be clear about safety issues and be strict in enforcing them.

Keep this meeting short, but don't skip over it.

12 Keys to Conducting Effective Practices

To this point you've learned about structuring your season and individual practices. The rest of this chapter is devoted to detailing 12 keys to running effective practices. Here are the keys:

1. Be prepared.
2. Set the stage.
3. Involve parents.
4. Be active.
5. Be active with a purpose.
6. Make it fun.
7. Provide instruction.
8. Give feedback.
9. Be encouraging and supportive.

10. Promote teamwork and camaraderie.

11. Discipline players as necessary.

12. Wrap up the practice.

1. Be Prepared

Sixty minutes—or however long you have for practice—goes by quickly. If you go into practice unprepared, it will go by inefficiently, too.

A little preparation can go a long way. Plan your practice, know what you need to teach, how you want to teach it, which stations you want to run, and which drills or games you want to use to help your players practice their skills. Choose effective drills and games to maximize the learning experience. Be prepared to instruct, give feedback, and provide encouragement.

That doesn't mean you can't adjust or deviate from your plan. It means you have a plan you can adjust as you need to.

2. Set the Stage

You need to not only have a plan, but also let your players in on that plan. It helps them focus when they know what they're going to practice that day. Let them know the purpose of each practice and the purpose of each drill or game at the practice stations.

How you approach the practice greatly influences your players. If you are cavalier or seemingly uncaring about what happens at practice, your players will follow suit. If you are focused and positive and have a purpose in mind, your players will be more tuned in to the drills and games.

Another way you set the stage is in teaching skills. Don't simply teach the mechanics; let players know why they need to perform the skill and in what type of situation they will be called upon to perform it in a game. You'll learn more about this in Chapter 6, "Player Development."

3. Involve Parents

Studies show that the more parents are involved in their kids' education, the better their kids do. This shouldn't be too surprising.

Parental involvement has the same effect on youth sport programs, too. But some coaches ward off parents, discouraging their participation. Why? Perhaps because the coaches fear they will lose control of the team when other adults step in or the coaches are concerned that their own lack of knowledge or coaching ability will be revealed. And then there are the few bad-apple parents who are know-it-alls or poor sports or who *do* want to impose their own will at practice. Coaches already have plenty to contend with and can't be blamed for not wanting to deal with this type of parent.

But coaches who steer clear of parental involvement miss out on the advantages that can come with involving them. Here are a few of the roles parents can serve:

- **Official or unofficial assistant coaches**—It's extremely helpful to have at least one assistant coach. As noted earlier, it's also helpful to have an adult, whether you call him or her an assistant coach or a parent aid or whatever, to supervise each station you run at practice. They can even help you instruct, if they know the skill and know how to teach it.

- **Drink and snack providers**—Set up a rotation for parents to provide drinks and snacks for games.

- **Special-event planners**—Ask a parent to organize any special event—a pizza party or swimming party—held during the season or for a postseason celebration.

tip

Some parents want to help but can't do so at every practice or game. Make it easy for these parents to help by setting up a parent helper rotation. Come up with the ways you need help, find out how many parents are willing to provide that type of help, and set up a rotation for practices and games, so the burden is light and shared.

4. Be Active

When you use simultaneous stations, kids are active. Kids can't improve if they have to wait for 14 teammates to attempt a pass or shot or tackle before they get a chance. Keep things moving at practice.

5. Be Active with a Purpose

But don't mistake movement and action with purpose. Kids standing around in practice doing nothing is not good; nor is kids bouncing all around the field like balls in a pinball machine with no purpose at all.

When you have prepared for the practice and have set the stage for it and for the games and drills the players are getting ready to participate in, then the players' actions are guided by a unified purpose. And when they're guided by that purpose, they are better prepared to learn and hone their skills.

6. Make It Fun

You can have a plan, and you can have a purpose to that plan, but if the practice is dull and boring, filled with repetitive drills that don't seem connected to the actual sport of soccer, then you're in trouble. Kids won't pay attention, they won't learn, and they won't care because they're not having fun.

Remember in Chapter 1, "Your Coaching Approach," when you learned about the reasons kids play soccer? The biggest reason they play is that they want to have fun.

Your goal is to teach your players soccer. Their goal is to have fun. When you make your teaching fun, everyone wins.

How do you make practices fun? You've already read about the main way: Keep the kids active. But there's another ingredient, too.

That ingredient is this: Don't practice skills by doing boring, repetitive drills. Practice skills in game-like conditions. This makes it more exciting for your players—and when they need to perform those skills in real games, they'll be more apt to succeed because they've been executing in those same situations during practice. In addition, kids understand tactics much better when those tactics are introduced and practiced in the context of real-game situations.

Read more about this concept in the following sidebar, "Using Game-like Situations in Practice."

USING GAME-LIKE SITUATIONS IN PRACTICE

Consider ways you could teach how to pass. You could pair up players, set them 5–7 yards from each other, and have them pass the ball back and forth.

This is useful, and you can make it challenging by having kids try to make 10, 15, or 20 good passes in a row. They can also use this drill at home with a brother or sister.

And you can supplement that drill with a game-like drill as well. For instance, you could play a game of 4v2 keep-away, with the four on offense trying to keep the two defenders from stealing the ball. Give them a big enough area to move in—enough that the offensive players can move to open areas to receive passes—and see how many passes the offense can complete, or how long the offense can go, before the defense gains possession.

This is both game-like and fun. Players will be learning what they have to do to get open in real games, what kinds of passes they need to make, and how to receive the ball and maintain possession.

Be creative. Put kids in game-like situations for all the skills and tactics they practice. When you do, you're doing everyone—including yourself—a favor.

7. Provide Instruction

The next three items on this list—instruction, feedback, and encouragement—are foundational elements in coaching at practice and are closely, and often sequentially, related.

Most coaches realize that to run an effective practice they need to provide quality instruction for their players. But providing good instruction isn't necessarily easy; it's accomplished through a set of learned skills. You'll learn about how to be an effective instructor and teacher of skills in Chapter 6.

8. Give Feedback

After you instruct your players, your coaching duties have just begun. As your players practice the tactics and skills you've taught them, you need to observe their play, assess their technique and understanding, and give them feedback on anything they're doing wrong and on what they should do to improve. How to provide this feedback is also covered in Chapter 6.

9. Be Encouraging and Supportive

All players—from youth leagues through to professional leagues—need encouragement and support. Soccer is an easy game to learn but a challenging one to master. The skills are not easy to acquire and, even once acquired, they are not easy to consistently execute.

Your players will struggle with picking up the basic skills and with consistently executing them. All players will struggle to improve, regardless of their skill level. You need to nurture their improvement with encouragement and provide a supportive environment for them—and the practice field is the place where this happens. You'll learn specifics of how to provide this encouragement in Chapter 6.

10. Promote Teamwork and Camaraderie

Soccer is a team game. Goals and great saves grab attention, but a nifty pass at midfield, a well-executed give-and-go, and a well-timed tackle can be just as crucial to a game's outcome. Can a high-scoring forward win games all by himself?

The teams that win more often than not are generally more fundamentally sound than other teams. They defend well; they know how to control the ball; they attack well as a team, spreading out and hitting the open areas; they help out on defense as needed; and they make crisp passes and sure receptions. They know what to do with the ball and when to do it. All the players contribute to the win.

One of the joys of playing sports is the camaraderie players experience with their teammates. This occurs as players struggle together, as they pull for each other, as they go through wins and losses together, and as they exult over individual successes and encourage each other in individual failures, all the while reinforcing the notion that those individual successes and failures are all part of a team effort.

That's how the game and the relationships between players *should* be viewed, and that's the environment you should cultivate. Here are a couple of ideas for cultivating it:

- At the beginning of the season, you or a player's parents could host a pizza and movie night. The players could get together, eat pizza, and play games or watch a movie.

- At the end of each practice, say something positive about each player. Don't force this; it has to be sincere. If it's too much to say something about every player, single out half of them for compliments at one practice, and address the other half of the team at the end of the next practice. "Way to pass, Jake," "Nice tackling today, Ramon," and "You made some nice saves as goalkeeper today, Michelle," are examples of the things you might say. When players hear you say something good about everyone, most often for doing small things correctly, it reinforces the team concept.

- Set up a buddy system at practice. Pair up players at each practice and ask that each player pick out something good that his partner did during practice. Switch buddies at each practice so kids get used to encouraging and complimenting different teammates. Again, this exchange shouldn't be forced; emphasize that you want the players to look for good things their teammates do and encourage them to continue to improve.

The main point is to look for ways to emphasize the team aspects of the game and cultivate an environment in which the support and encouragement doesn't just flow from coach to players, but from player to player as well.

11. Discipline Players As Necessary

Part of running an effective practice is to take care of any discipline problems that arise, so they don't disrupt the practice.

Even when you conduct a practice that keeps the players active through fun and meaningful drills and games, some kids might misbehave. Here are some suggestions for dealing with different types of misbehavior:

- **Minor misbehavior**—Many times you can ignore minor misbehavior, so long as it doesn't disrupt the practice or distract others from hearing you or from practicing. Kids will sometimes clown around or goof off to draw attention; sometimes if you ignore that behavior, the child will stop it without being told to. If the child *doesn't* stop it and it becomes a distraction to others, you should put a stop to it.

- ■ **Disrespect**—When a player shows disrespect, either to you or to another player, don't let it pass. Use appropriate measures to stop the disrespect.

- ■ **Repeated misbehavior**—If a player is repeatedly misbehaving, even if it's minor misbehavior, you need to address this. Talk to the player, tell him what behavior you need from him and, if the misbehavior continues, punish him appropriately. You might also want to call his parents to let them know of the problem and work together to steer the child toward good behavior.

- ■ **Behavior that puts someone in danger**—You need to put an immediate stop to any behavior that puts someone in danger, and you need to discipline the misbehaving player accordingly.

When you do need to discipline players, do so consistently and impartially. Stick to what you say; if you tell them they will be disciplined for a certain type of behavior, and you don't follow through, you're in for trouble.

After you have disciplined a player, don't hold past misbehavior against that player. Also, never discipline a player for making a mistake, and don't use physical activity—such as running or doing pushups—as a form of punishment. That sends the message that physical activity is bad.

You shouldn't have to discipline your players too much—especially if you keep them engaged in fun activities throughout practice.

12. Wrap Up the Practice

Sixty minutes flies by, and most coaches want to squeeze as much practice as possible out of their time with their players. But it's helpful to take at least a few minutes to wrap up the practice with a brief meeting.

At this meeting, go over what went well, encourage your players (or have them encourage each other, using the buddy system as described earlier), talk about a few things they still need to work on or give constructive feedback based on what you observed in practice, and remind them of the next game or practice. Send the players off with an encouraging word and a smile.

And make sure you're the last to leave the practice field, so that you know every player got a ride home.

Then, go home yourself—and plan for your next great practice!

THE ABSOLUTE MINIMUM

This chapter was devoted to helping you construct season and practice plans and to knowing how to run effective practices. Among the key points were

- Make a season plan before your season begins so you can see the big picture of what you want to accomplish and plan to teach the skills and tactics in a logical order.

- Be willing to adjust your season plan as necessary, based on what your players need.

- Create a practice plan for each practice, one with a specific purpose. Don't forget to teach rules that are related to the skills and tactics you present in that practice.

- At your first practice, let your players know your goals for the season, your expectations of them, what they can expect from you, what the team rules are (as well as the consequences of breaking them), and what the basic practice structure will be.

- Run simultaneous stations in practice so your players are as active as possible. Develop these stations with players' safety in mind.

- Involve parents in running these stations and in other areas where you could use help.

- Focus these stations on fun game-like drills and activities. Players who learn skills in the context of how they should be executed in games are best prepared to execute those skills properly in real games.

- Provide skill instruction, feedback on performance, and encouragement. Cultivate a team atmosphere that promotes camaraderie.

- Discipline players as necessary, following through in appropriate ways that steer the players toward better behavior.

In This Chapter

- The process for teaching skills and tactics
- Six keys to error correction

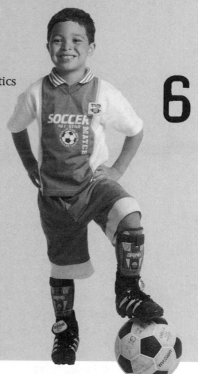

6

Player Development

Practice time is all about your players learning and developing the skills and tactics they need to successfully execute in games. And that means you have to be a good teacher, a keen observer, a patient guide, and an encouraging critic.

Sound like a lot? It is, but you can learn how to provide this instruction and guidance. And it's critical that you do because, without it, your players will not fully develop their talents and both you and they will be frustrated.

So, get ready to learn how to teach skills and tactics, how to observe your players and give them the feedback they need, and how to correct errors. In Chapter 11, "Games and Drills," you'll find games and drills you can use to teach your players the skills and tactics they need to know.

The Process for Teaching Skills and Tactics

"Hey, this skill is simple. Even I can do it, and I'm not that good. Why can't they do it?"

"I told them how to dribble. I was concise, clear, and to the point. Why aren't they doing it right?"

"I spent 10 minutes going into detail on how to tackle, but I might as well have been talking to myself, from all the good it did."

Those are among the comments of new coaches, especially if they haven't been in a position to teach before. In the first case, the skill is only simple to the coach, who has likely performed it before. It's not that simple to his players. In the second case, kids need more than an explanation of the skill; they need to see it performed as well. And in the third case, don't mistake the practice field for the lecture hall. Kids don't need a long-winded speech about every minor detail of the skill as it is performed. If you provide one, be prepared for your players to doze off—just as you probably would have at their age.

What *do* your players need? They need you to set the stage for their learning. They need you to show and tell them how to perform the skill or tactic. They need, of course, to practice the skill or tactic. And they need your feedback as they practice.

Set the Stage

The players have just finished warm-ups and Coach Jarvis is ready to practice tackling. He calls the players over to him, but Jake and Deon don't hear their coach because they're talking as they warm up.

"All right, guys, we're going to practice a little defense," Coach Jarvis says. Then the coach notices Jake and Deon and calls them over. As they make their way over, Coach Jarvis says, "Let's split into three groups of four players each, two balls for each group. All right?"

If Coach Jarvis were playing goalkeeper, he would have just let three straight shots go through his legs. That is, he made three mistakes in setting the stage for this skill instruction:

1. He didn't make sure all his players were listening to him before he began giving instructions.
2. He didn't tell them precisely what they were going to practice.
3. He didn't tell them when or how they would use this skill—whatever it was—in a game.

Why are these things important? Let's look at each issue.

Players' Focus

Coach Jarvis began explaining, in rather cryptic fashion, what the players were going to do before all the players were even within earshot. Even if Coach Jarvis had explained it well, Jake and Deon would have been in the dark about what they were going to be doing.

When you explain a skill or drill to your team, first make sure you have everyone's attention, so practice won't be slowed down as you find yourself explaining things two or three times (see Figure 6.1). Getting your players' attention can sometimes be challenging because two of the main reasons most kids plays sports is they want to have fun and they want to hang out with their friends. Put those two together, and add in other external and internal distractions, and coaches quickly find that they can't assume their players will always be ready to give them their full attention.

> **tip**
>
> To get your players' attention, call them together and make eye contact with each one. If some aren't looking at you, call their names so you make eye contact. Wait until the players are quiet and attentive. If this doesn't happen within a few moments, ask them to stop talking, look at you, and give you their full attention. Don't go on until they do so.

FIGURE 6.1

Get your players' attention before you explain a skill.

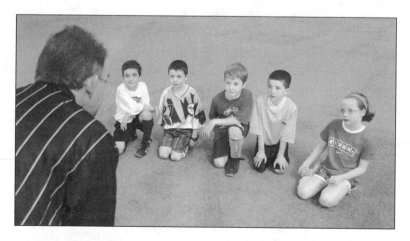

Name That Skill

When you have their attention, identify the skill or tactic you're going to teach. For example, Coach Jarvis should have said something like, "Today we're going to learn how to execute a block tackle."

Why? For a couple of reasons. First, it gives the players a reference point later. When Coach Jarvis talks about block tackles, his players will know what he's referring to. For another, it often helps kids get a mental picture of what they're going to be doing. Mainly, though, it helps avoid confusion later. "Practice a little defense" covers a wide variety of skills; referring to this won't help your players recall anything. "Making block tackles" is explicit and clear and will help them recall the skills involved.

Skill Context

During a league game, Jason receives a pass just past midfield, dribbles for a few steps, and then fires a long shot that is well off target and doesn't even reach the goal. The next time down the field, he does the same thing, firing away at the goal when he has no chance of scoring and when he should be looking to pass the ball to a teammate.

At halftime, as other players are getting a drink, you ask Jason why he was firing such long shots. "Because you told us the only way we can score is to shoot," he replies.

This is true; you *did* say that. But you didn't mean for players to take shots from midfield. You meant to say shoot as soon as you have a good opportunity to score and look to create those opportunities as often as possible.

Many coaches do well in getting their players' attention and in naming a skill before they begin to teach it, but they don't realize the importance of putting that skill into context for the players. *You* might recognize a good scoring opportunity, but your players might not. And if they don't, chances are they won't successfully execute when those opportunities arise.

To help them understand, you could ask a few questions like, "Who can tell me what offside is?" "What should a player do if she finds herself in danger of being offside?" If you receive a correct answer, make sure everyone heard it and understands it before moving on. If you're not sure whether everyone heard or understands, or if no one gave a correct answer, give a brief, clear answer yourself—something like, "Offside is when your teammate passes you the ball and you're on the offensive end of the field and only the goalie is between you and the goal. If a teammate is in an offside position, don't pass the ball to her. If you're the one in the offside position, don't take part in the play. Run to the sideline or to a point where another defender besides the goalie is between you and the goal. That way you won't be called for offside."

Don't take long with this explanation, but do be clear about when the situation comes up and what its tactical importance is to the team. Let your players know how the team benefits when the skill or tactic is correctly executed.

> **note**
>
> One of the joys of coaching is when you see your players respond correctly in a situation without telling them what to do. When you put tactics and skills in context of how they're used in a game, your players will learn not just the tactic or skill, but also the game itself.

Show and Tell

Naming the skill and putting it in context should take just a few moments. The next step, "show and tell," will take a little longer.

Some inexperienced coaches make the mistake of *telling* their players how to perform a skill but not *showing* them how. A verbal explanation isn't enough. Neither is just a visual demonstration. If you briefly explain the skill as you demonstrate it, it should sink in (see Figure 6.2).

For example, in teaching how to receive a pass, tell your players to get in front of the ball, watch it, cushion it, and keep it near their bodies—and demonstrate this as you tell them. The visual demonstration is vital to their comprehension.

tip

If you're a coach who hasn't played soccer before, don't panic. Just recruit a skilled high school player to demonstrate the skill. High school athletes tend to enjoy helping out in such a way.

FIGURE 6.2

Show the skill as you explain it.

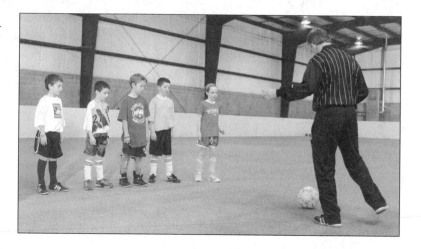

Here are a few pointers on what to say about a skill and how to demonstrate it.

What to say:

- Briefly and clearly explain the technique. You should be able to explain the technique for most skills in no more than a minute or two.

- Use language your players understand.

- Ask your players how they are going to perform the skill after you're finished explaining and demonstrating it, to see if they understand what to do.

tip

Watch for comprehension on your players' faces as you explain a skill. If you see a confused look, clear up the confusion before you have the players practice the skill.

What to show:

- Perform the skill as you talk your way through it.
- Show the skill a few times.
- If necessary, use an assistant coach, a parent, or a player to help you demonstrate a skill. You might need to use someone else either to show correct form or to show how two players execute a tactic.
- Break a skill down in parts, showing each part first and then showing the complete skill without a break. For example, on receiving a pass, show how to get in front of the ball as it comes to you. Then show how to watch the ball all the way. Then show how to cushion the ball and keep it near your body. Finally, show the complete skill all at once.

Practice the Skill

After you've introduced a skill and shown and told your players how to perform it, have them practice the skill in game-like situations. Use drills or games that simulate the experiences they will have in real games and observe their techniques.

Here are suggestions for constructing games and drills that simulate real-game situations and maximize player participation:

- Construct most games with the simultaneous-station idea in mind. That means you'll generally have four or five players per game or drill. This allows more opportunities for each player to practice the skill.
- You can also inject some controlled scrimmages during the latter part of the practice, in which you set up plays and have each team execute the plays, keeping score based on their successful executions.
- Focus the action on the skill you want your players to practice, with as little other action surrounding that skill execution as possible. Take care, though, to keep the action realistic, not cutting off too much.
- As noted in Chapter 5, "Practice Plans," you should make the games and drills fun. Score them in some way, make them competitive, or add a twist to them while maintaining their realism.
- Construct each game around a singular, clear purpose. Directly tie in to the purpose the successful execution of the skill or tactic.
- Consider ways to make the games a little easier for less talented players and a little harder for more skilled players.
- Make the games simple to explain and understand. You don't want to spend 5 minutes explaining the game and spend additional time reexplaining it as the players play.

Be sure to see the sample games and drills in Chapter 11 for offensive skills, defensive skills, and tactics.

Provide Feedback

As players take part in a drill or game, practicing the skill or tactic you've just taught them, observe their execution and be ready to provide feedback to help them correct errors and improve their play. In this section, you learn about feedback content, timing, whether you should alter your feedback for athletes of varying abilities, and what to do for the kids who just don't seem to get it.

Feedback Content

Focus most of your feedback on the players' attempts to execute the skill or tactic you just taught. Don't overload them with feedback as they practice, but do give your attackers coaching cues, such as "Spread out the attack," "Look for your open teammate," or "Follow through on your shots." Similar cues to your defenders might be "Keep in position," "Go for the tackle," and "Watch the middle." These comments are short enough not to distract them and should serve as reminders of the technique you just taught.

However, that doesn't mean you can't provide some feedback concerning related skills. Maybe you just taught the technique for marking and now you're conducting a marking drill or game. As the players take part in the game, you see that they are having trouble with basic dribbling skills, so you provide the same type of coaching cues to remind them of proper dribbling technique: "Keep it close," "Use both sides of the foot," or "Shield the ball."

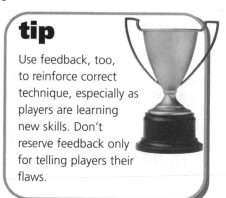

tip

Use feedback, too, to reinforce correct technique, especially as players are learning new skills. Don't reserve feedback only for telling players their flaws.

Feedback Timing

In most cases, the best time to give feedback is as soon as you see something you should comment on, either affirming correct technique or helping a player improve incorrect technique. Many times, as mentioned, you can use coaching cues to remind players of correct technique; you can give these cues as they are participating in the drill or game without stopping the flow.

You can also provide feedback at the end of the drill or game or at the end of practice, especially if what you have to say applies to multiple players.

If you have feedback that really applies only to one player, in addition to giving feedback on the spot, you can also draw that player aside after the drill or at the end of practice and give him your feedback.

If several of your players are having difficulty performing the skill you just taught and they appear not to know how to go about it, you need to stop the action and reteach the skill. There was a disconnection between your teaching and their learning, and you need to teach the skill in a way that is clear to them—or ask yourself whether the skill is too advanced for their ability level. If that's the case, perhaps you need to keep your players focused on refining the fundamental skills.

Altering Your Feedback

Theo, Albert, and Chris are three of the players who play forward for you.

Theo is a superb forward. He has a knack for being in the right place at the right time, has a strong and accurate shot, and is a great passer. He also has above-average ball control skills. Theo is a sharp kid, a "quiet leader" type who's always focused and tough internally. He doesn't like to make mistakes, of course, but he shakes them off when he does.

Albert has some talent, but he is a year younger than Theo, is less mature, and is inconsistent with his mechanics. He appears lackadaisical at times and often is not in the best position to receive a pass or take a shot.

Chris has limited talent, but he loves the game, tries hard, and gets down on himself when he doesn't make plays he thinks he should have. Chris is the least-skilled of the three, although he's more consistent than Albert.

Do you provide the same type of feedback to Theo, Albert, and Chris? Let's say that on the exact same type of two-on-two situation near the goal, your three forwards do this:

- Theo gets free with a good head fake, receives a pass, and immediately scores.

- Albert is momentarily open, but doesn't move as his defender comes over to defend him. A pass to him is intercepted. Albert shrugs and watches his defender move down the field with the ball.

- Chris does his best to get open for a pass, but his defender is quick and stays with him. Chris finally does manage to get open; he receives a pass and takes a shot that is easily stopped by the goalkeeper. Chris is upset with himself that he didn't score.

With Theo, you tell him, "Way to go!" But what about Albert and Chris? Their outcome was similar—they didn't score—but you feel Albert should have tried harder to get open and get a shot off but just gave up on it, while Chris tried his hardest and did get a shot off but just couldn't score.

You should applaud Chris for his efforts and encourage him. In Albert's case, you might say, "Albert, you need to keep moving to stay open! Lose your defender! You can do it!"

The point is that you will be giving feedback on effort and mental approach as well as physical technique. You will be giving feedback to players with a lot of talent, players who have minimal talent, and players who vary in their desires for the game and their emotional makeup.

Shape your feedback to best help the player improve his or her abilities to play the game. Don't panic; this doesn't mean you have to have a different approach for every player. It just means you need to consider what type of feedback will best help the player improve.

Theo and Chris likely won't need any encouragement from you to give it their all. They *will* likely need feedback on technique, but you shouldn't expect Chris to perform at the same level as Theo, so your feedback will be tempered by that and by your understanding that he's hard on himself. You want to focus your feedback on the technical aspects of their play and give all your players—especially those who, like Chris, are hard on themselves—plenty of encouragement.

As you get to know your players, this tailoring of feedback becomes relatively simple. For now, be aware that, just as your players are individuals, you should shape your feedback according to their individual needs, all with the same end goal in mind: to help them improve their skills.

If at First a Player Doesn't Succeed...

...*don't* ask her to just "try, try again," even though that's how the saying goes. Instead, ask yourself why the player is failing.

Why ask this question? Because a player can make a mistake for many reasons, and the reason should affect how you respond. Here are some of the reasons:

- The player doesn't know the correct technique.
- She knows the correct technique but doesn't understand the rules or the specific strategy called for.
- She doesn't appear to be giving her full effort.
- She is too anxious about her performance.

Let's consider how you should respond in each situation.

If a player is making mistakes because she doesn't know the correct technique, she doesn't need your encouragement; she needs your instruction on the mechanics of the skill.

If a player knows the correct technique but makes a mistake because she's not sure what to do, you need to clarify the rules or explain the strategy called for in that situation.

If a player makes a mistake or doesn't make a play because of a lack of desire or effort, you need to talk privately with the player and find out why she is giving less than full effort. You should work with the player to eradicate the problem and encourage her to give full effort at all times, both for herself and for her teammates.

If a player is making mistakes because she is overanxious about her performance, you should talk with this player privately and help her put her performance in perspective. If the anxiety continues, consider moving her to a different position on the field, with the intent of taking pressure off of her. Help her focus on the technical, physical aspects of the game.

What if a player knows the correct technique, knows the rules and strategies involved, is giving full effort, and isn't overly anxious about her performance but she still makes lots of mistakes?

This youngster needs two things: practice and encouragement. Provide all the opportunities you can for her in practice, and suggest to her parents that they might work with her at home on her skills.

Six Keys to Error Correction

You've heard the saying, "Practice makes perfect." Well, if practice made perfect, then professional soccer players would never make a mistake. And while practice certainly helps players improve, you will have plenty of technical flaws and other types of errors to correct. Here are six keys to correcting errors:

1. Be encouraging.
2. Be honest.
3. Be specific.
4. Reinforce correct technique.
5. Explain why the error happened.
6. Watch for comprehension.

Let's consider each key.

Be Encouraging

Players are usually discouraged when they make a mistake. They need to be corrected, but they also need to be encouraged.

Look for something you can praise, even as you prepare to correct the player. Commend him for his effort. Acknowledge something that he did correctly: "That's the way to go after the ball, John." And after you have corrected his technique, end with a smile and a word of encouragement.

Be Honest

Be encouraging, yes, but don't be dishonest. Don't say, "Nice pass, Nick!" if Nick's pass leaves much to be desired. False praise isn't going to help Nick; honesty and correction are.

And don't falsely praise some inconsequential thing, just to give some praise. Kids see through that, and if they know you're not leveling with them, they will be insulted and might question more legitimate comments you make. For example, let's say a midfielder deftly dribbles beyond a defender and then makes a hard, sharp pass that is well off the mark and goes out of bounds, untouched. You shout, "Way to zing the ball up field!" The player will either think you're making fun of him or know you're reaching for a compliment because he passed the ball poorly. Even if he kicked it hard, the result was a mistake and nothing about the pass could be realistically complimented. You *could*, however, compliment the player for his footwork and ball control and then tell him how to correct his passing.

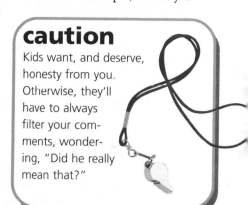

caution

Kids want, and deserve, honesty from you. Otherwise, they'll have to always filter your comments, wondering, "Did he really mean that?"

Be Specific

When you correct faulty technique, be specific. During goalkeeping practice, don't say, "Come on, Andi! We need you to defend better than that!" That doesn't help Andi know what she's doing incorrectly. Rather, say, "Andi, when you're catching a ball in the air, give with it a little. Move back with it, and use your fingertips, not your palms, to catch it. You can do it."

Focus your correction on the technical aspects the player needs to change, being clear and specific in your comments. Keep your feedback short and precise, and remember to demonstrate the correct action to reinforce your verbal message (see Figure 6.3).

Reinforce Correct Technique

In a drill that focuses on receiving passes with the thigh, Ben keeps bouncing the ball off his knee, causing it to bounce far from him.

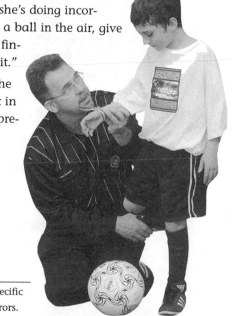

FIGURE 6.3

Be clear and specific in correcting errors.

Some inexperienced coaches would take the pains to show Ben just what he did wrong: His thigh wasn't parallel to the ground; he brought his knee up rapidly at the last instant to make his thigh parallel; he was too far from the ball and kept receiving it on his knee.

And they would be wasting their time.

Why? Because Ben already knows he used incorrect technique. You don't need to demonstrate what he did wrong; he already attempted to receive the ball that way. He needs to see what he *should* do.

Many times, even if you say, "Don't do it this way," or "Here's what you did wrong," as you show the incorrect technique, the player does not hear the message or the incorrect technique is reinforced in his mind's eye because he's seeing it all over again.

Simply show him how to correctly perform the technique, tell him what to do, and let him try it again.

Explain Why the Error Happened

Sometimes kids don't understand what they're doing wrong. You can briefly explain it, without demonstrating the incorrect technique. This explanation can help them understand what they're doing wrong and, as you tell and show them how to execute the skill correctly, they are more likely to get it if they understand what to change.

For example, if a goalkeeper has trouble stopping shots that are at an angle from the goal, tell her she's having trouble because she's not cutting off the angle of the shot. Then tell and show her how to cut off the angle of the shot.

Most often, however, your players will not need much of an explanation for why they committed the mistake. Focus most of your time on explaining and demonstrating correct technique.

Watch for Comprehension

Earlier you read about the need to watch for comprehension on your players' faces as you teach them a new skill. You need to watch for this same comprehension as you correct their technique, too.

Look for understanding in your players' eyes and if there's any doubt, ask them, "Do you understand what I mean?" If they don't, couch your verbal message differently, making sure your demonstration of the technique is clear as well.

The effectiveness of your correction is not based on how clear your message is to you; it's based on how well it's received by your players.

THE ABSOLUTE MINIMUM

This chapter focused on your approach to teaching skills and tactics and correcting errors. Key points to remember include

- Remember the method to teaching skills: Set the stage for your players' learning; use a show-and-tell approach to teaching; practice the skill; and provide feedback.

- In setting the stage, make sure your players are listening, name the skill, and put it in context for your players so they can see how they will use it in a game and how correct execution of the skill will benefit the team.

- In the show-and-tell phase, briefly and clearly explain and demonstrate the skill. Watch for player comprehension as you do this, and be ready to clear up any confusion.

- Break down a skill in parts, showing each individual part alone, and then perform the entire skill at once.

- Provide clear feedback to help players improve their skills.

- Consider reasons players are making mistakes and tailor your feedback accordingly. Sometimes they might not know how to perform the skill and need skill instruction; at other times they might understand how to perform the skill but need help improving their mechanics. They also might not understand the rules or strategies that relate to the situation.

- When correcting errors, keep these six keys in mind: Be encouraging; be honest; be specific; reinforce correct technique; explain why the error happened; and watch for comprehension.

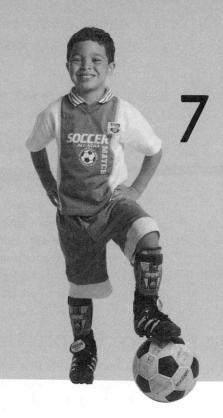

7

GAME TIME!

Parents, grandparents, and siblings of players begin to arrive at the field. The players arrive singly and in pairs, looking crisp and sharp in their uniforms. The referee is on hand, and the field is freshly mown and green. As your players warm up, you can see the excitement in their faces.

A few butterflies stir to life in your stomach. For every butterfly fluttering in your stomach, you figure there must be a dozen in your players' bellies. Anticipation, hope, anxiety, and joy intermingle in the air. In a few minutes, the players will stride onto the field and the game will begin.

There's nothing like game time, nothing like that first kickoff, releasing the tension that has been building since the first players arrived for warm-ups.

Playing games is really what it's all about. Kids come to practice to learn and hone skills with one purpose in mind: to play as well as possible during games. It takes planning and expertise to make practices fun, but playing league games is *inherently* fun, and the main reason that most kids sign up to play.

So far, you've learned to apply the keys to coaching to your practices. In this chapter you learn to apply those keys before, during, and after games. What should you communicate to your players at the practice before a game? When the game rolls around, do you change your approach to coaching in any way? How should you rotate players in and out? How much teaching and error correction should you do during a game? How much strategy should you employ during a game? What should you tell players before and after a game? For the answers to these and many similar questions, read on.

The Practice Before the Game

For the most part, the practice immediately preceding a game will not differ from any other practice. But there are a few things you need to discuss with your players, including the game particulars and the team's tactical focus for the game.

Game Particulars

At the end of the practice, remind the players of the game time, the field location, and what time you want them to arrive at the field to warm up. Tell them to arrive 20 minutes before the game so they have enough time to warm up. Remind them to wear their team uniforms and bring their water bottles.

Many games are played around dinnertime or shortly after. Give your players some guidance on what to eat, what not to eat, and how soon before a game they should eat. See the following sidebar, "Fueling Up," for guidelines on what players should eat and drink before, during, and after games.

tip

If a game is canceled, a phone tree is a great way to get the word our quickly while not taking a lot of your own time. Just set up a system so you're sure that everyone is called.

FUELING UP

It's 20 minutes before game time. Do you know what's in your players' stomachs? Whatever it is, they will use it as the fuel in their tanks for the game.

Hopefully, their fuel doesn't consist of a big steak dinner or a couple of fast-food burgers lathered in "special" (read: *fat-laden*) sauce, with a large order of fries, washed down with a soft drink.

Why? Because foods high in fat take longer to digest. Your players should have easily digested food in their stomachs, so their energy goes toward playing rather than digesting. The carbonation in soft drinks can cause indigestion, and the sugar content results in a rise in blood insulin levels, which can make players tired. Tell your players not to have soft drinks within a few hours of a game.

That doesn't mean they should show up empty-stomached. That's like taking off on a drive with your gas tank all but dry.

Players should have something light and digestible an hour or two before the game—a bagel or toast and a little fruit would be good, though a lot of fruit can cause gastrointestinal stress. Some cereal to tide them over until after the game works, too.

If they have time, they can eat a light meal two to three hours before the game. This meal should be high in carbohydrates and low in fat.

As for fluids, players should drink water before, during, and after a game. Sports drinks are good, too, and provide the added benefit of replacing minerals and electrolytes lost through exercise and sweat. Players should drink two or three cups of water or sports drink (24–30 ounces) within two hours of a game and drink about 8 ounces of fluid every 20 minutes during a game.

Game Focus

Your team's tactical focus might consist solely of executing the fundamentals well—and if your team does that, it has an excellent chance of winning. Especially at younger levels of play, there isn't much need for intricate tactics; you want your players to simply focus on executing the individual skills well.

At the younger levels, your strategy should be easily remembered, with much or all of it becoming part of your season-long mantra: "Spread the offense out. Make good passes. Control the ball. Mark your man on defense."

> **tip**
>
> Don't just dictate team strategy for older players; ask for their input. This helps them to consider their strengths and the strategies that would help them win. It also results in them perhaps more fully buying into the strategies because they had a part in designing them.

If you are coaching older or more experienced players, however, you can and should consider your tactical approach to the game. This approach hinges on your players' strengths and abilities and on the opponent you're facing.

Here are some of the team tactical approaches you might consider:

- **Use your ball-control skills to maintain possession**—You can't score if you don't have the ball, and you can't maintain possession of the ball if you don't have ball-control skills. If you can maintain possession, you can continue to push forward, putting pressure on the defense and looking for the right openings.

■ **Use your passing and receiving skills to penetrate the defense**—A good passing and receiving team is a constant threat because it can quickly gain an advantage.

■ **Spread out the offense**—At younger levels, it's common to see swarms of players around the ball, like villagers surrounding Frankenstein. The poor ball doesn't have a chance. Neither does the offense because, instead of spreading out the attack, they have all surrounded the ball and are trying to group-kick it. The team that can spread out, find the holes and seams, and use the field is light years ahead of the game.

■ **Help out in defending the most dangerous opponents**—Often a team has one or two players who are more dangerous than their teammates on offense. When you can recognize the main threats and place your emphasis on defending them (by putting your best defenders on them and instructing your other players to be ready to help out), you increase your chances of effectively defending against the opponents' main threats.

Before the Game

Arrive about 30 minutes before game time, if possible. Use the 10 minutes or so that you have before your players arrive to check the field. Just as you do before practices, look for broken glass, potholes, or any other hazards and take care of them if you can. If you can't, talk with the opposing coach and referees about how to ensure players' safety, and report the problem to your league administrator after the game.

In addition to checking the field, you have two other duties to tend to before the game begins: making sure your team warms up properly and giving your players a few pearls of wisdom before they take to the field.

Team Warm-up

This is simple enough, and players should know the routine from practice. They need to jog a few minutes, stretch, and do some passing and dribbling drills. Make sure your goalkeeper gets some practice stopping shots, too.

In "Player Substitutions" later in this chapter, you'll consider options in rotating players in and out of the lineup, rotating players at various positions, and dealing with playing time issues.

Last-minute Words

As noted in Chapter 3, "Communication Keys," you don't need to fire up your troops with a dramatic pep talk. But you do need to help them prepare to compete, and a few well-chosen words before the game can do just that.

Remind them to focus on the basics and to execute the fundamental skills and tactics they have been practicing. Go over any particular strategies or game plans you discussed in the previous practice. You might also note how you will substitute players in, although you don't necessarily need to divulge this. Sometimes, however, it's easy enough to let players know the general approach to when and how they will be subbed in, and this can help them get mentally prepared.

Above all, tell them to play hard and have fun.

Your talk might go something like this: "Just focus on what we've been working on: ball control, good passing, spreading out the offense, and solid marking. Let's play hard, play smart, and have fun. Are you ready?"

This will help focus your players on the fundamentals, remind them of the game plan, and help them keep the big picture in mind.

During the Game

You know your role as coach at practice and how to plan for practices and run them effectively.

But what, if anything, changes for you during games? Does your coaching role change? Is there a subtle shift in your approach? Do you do the same amount of coaching and the same type of coaching? How do you respond to players' mistakes, and how do you plan to rotate your players in and out?

This section takes a look at your role as coach during the game, providing strategies and tips to help you effectively guide your players throughout the contest.

Your Approach to the Game

During every practice, your focus is on helping your players acquire and develop the physical skills, tactical abilities, and mental approach and understanding to do what? To compete, with the goal of winning clearly in mind. Winning is the common goal of every team. Your job is to prepare your players in a way that puts them in a position to compete and to win.

Your job is also, as stated in Chapter 1, "Your Coaching Approach," to not overemphasize winning. Or, more directly put, to emphasize player development over winning. Of course, when you emphasize this development, you increase your chances of winning, so you're not working against yourself or your players here.

This all sounds so much easier than it really is. The pressure to win is enormous, and the inclination among players and coaches alike is to define themselves according to their win-loss record or personal achievements.

If you approach the game in a way that reinforces that winning-is-everything mentality in players' minds, you are doing them a disservice. If your coaching decisions reflect your concern first for your players and their development, and then your desire to win, you have the right approach. But you have to consciously go into each game with this mindset because the common mindset runs contrary to this.

Other considerations in your approach include how much coaching you do, what type of coaching you provide, and how you address or correct errors during games. Let's examine these issues one at a time.

How Much Coaching?

How much coaching you do during a game depends on what your players need. You don't want to over-coach, and you don't want to under-coach.

Some of the signs of over-coaching include

- You prepare and rehearse a 5-minute pep talk aimed solely at "firing up" the troops.
- You never stop talking throughout the game. When on offense you tell your players how to attack, and when on defense you tell your players who to mark and what to watch for. The game is a running monologue for you.
- When a player makes a mistake, you take him out and give him detailed skill instruction on the sideline.
- You spend hours analyzing your team's statistics after games.
- You get all over the 16-year-old referee because you think he missed a call.
- You send a scout to watch your next opponent's practice.

Almost as bad as over-coaching is under-coaching. Some of the signs of under-coaching include

- You don't tell your players what to focus on before the game begins; you simply show up, wish your players "Good luck," and settle in to watch the game.
- You don't provide any brief coaching tips or cues to your players.
- When a player asks you for some specific guidance, you just clap your hands and say, "Do your best."
- You give no encouragement to your players.

- One of your players is losing her cool and is on the borderline of getting a red card, and you don't intervene.

- One of your players is upset about a mistake he has made, and he is in tears on the sideline as you stand, passive and mute, a few feet away.

There are some extreme examples in both of those lists, but they aren't so extreme, unfortunately, as to be rare. What you should aim for is something that falls between over- and under-coaching. What's the right amount of coaching in youth soccer? Here are seven keys to coaching effectively during games:

- **Help your players get mentally prepared**—Remind them of their focus for the game and of any game plan that you devised in the previous practice. Keep them zoned in on properly executing the fundamentals. They will have nervous energy; you need to help them direct and expend that energy in ways that will help them compete well.

- **Provide tactical direction**—Briefly guide your players in the appropriate tactics as situations arise. Don't expect them to automatically know what to do in each situation.

- **Be involved, and be encouraging**—Part of being involved happens as you provide that tactical direction. Stay in the game mentally and emotionally. Encourage your players, and foster that same type of support among the players themselves.

- **Give technique tips and reminders**—Don't go into full-blown, detailed instruction on skills; save that for the next practice if you see that players are not executing correctly. Giving too much instruction during a game takes a player's focus off the game itself. But *do* give technique tips and reminders, cues that will help them remember what you taught them in practice: "Use the outside of your foot!"; "Follow through!"; or "Cushion the ball!" These technique tips should be enough to remind them of the more complete instruction you gave at previous practices.

> **tip**
>
> To provide helpful tips that don't distract your players, keep them short, clear, specific, and related directly to what you have previously taught.

- **Let the players play**—Guide your players, yes, but don't be like a puppeteer, with invisible strings attached to them, prompting their every move. It's your duty to teach them the skills and tactics and to let them experience the game as they compete against other teams. You coach and direct during games, but not with such a heavy hand that your players can't, or don't want to, think for themselves. Part of the joy for the players is learning how to perform and make decisions in games. Beyond ensuring that all your players get in the game, don't make numerous personnel moves, and don't constantly shout out instructions. Keep in the game, give players technique tips and encouragement, and let them play.

- **Tend to your players' needs**—Letting your players play doesn't mean you don't tend to their needs. Remind them before the game of your tactical approach or game plan. Give them coaching tips, support, and encouragement. If a player is disconsolate, tend to him; if a player twists an ankle, tend to her. Provide general direction throughout the game. And supply one more thing, which is the final item in this list.

- **Help your players keep the proper perspective**—Many coaches provide essentially everything their players need, except for this last item: keeping the game in perspective. These coaches build up each game as if it's the Major League Soccer championship game and celebrate wins excessively, while moping or grousing about the referees in defeat. Their players, of course, tend to take their cues from these coaches. The players make more of victories than they should and are poor sports or depressed in defeat, sulking or obsessing over a play they could have made that might have turned the game around.

  Don't do this to your players! Don't make more of a victory than it is because then kids get too wrapped up in the game's outcome, which they can't control. Keep them focused on their performances, which they *can* control. Even in victory, there are things to improve, and even in defeat, there are successes to be found. Help your players enjoy the game, to play it hard and as well as they can, and to learn from both wins and losses, while keeping both in proper perspective. It is, after all, a game. And it should be left on the field, win or lose. Young hearts and minds shouldn't labor long over a loss, and young heads shouldn't become so large after a win that players have difficulty pulling their shirts off when they get home.

Positive Coaching

Imagine Coach Swanson, in irritation or anger, shouting these comments during a game, for everyone (his players, opposing players, and fans) to hear:

"Come on, Nathan! You should have stopped that shot! How many times have I told you to stay down on shots!"

"Lucas! Do you call that marking?"

"Ann, you have to go after that ball! You let the other team get it because you waited for it to come to you!"

Chances are pretty good that Nathan, Lucas, and Ann will play the rest of the game with one eye on their coach, hoping not to make another play that draws Coach Swanson's ire or derogatory comments.

There's something about public humiliation that makes kids tentative.

Yet way too many coaches publicly humiliate their players, either consciously or unconsciously. These are the same coaches who attach too much importance to winning, who conveniently forget to put in their least-skilled players (or try to hide them in the field for a short time), and who grouse all game long at the referees.

It would have been far more appropriate if Coach Swanson had taken Nathan, Lucas, and Ann aside—not in a huge public display, but privately, perhaps at the quarter break—and calmly given each child the brief technique tip that he or she needed, along with an encouraging pat on the back before sending him or her back out on the field.

Look to build up your players, not tear them down. Teach in a positive manner, and keep control of your own emotions. Keep your comments focused on the techniques players need to improve, delivering them in a way that lets players know you are on their side. Remind them of times in the past when they performed the skill well. Help them to see themselves successfully performing it, and show by your words and body language that you believe they can do it again.

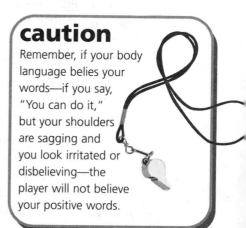

caution

Remember, if your body language belies your words—if you say, "You can do it," but your shoulders are sagging and you look irritated or disbelieving—the player will not believe your positive words.

Minimal Error Correction

Your players are going to make mistakes. In most cases, you'll have multiple errors in a game that you will need to address. So much of coaching is helping players correct mistakes. So, how should you approach this duty during games?

First, note the types of mistakes that are made by more than one player. You should address the necessary skill execution for the entire team in your next practice.

Second, note mistakes made by individual players. Perhaps Bobby has a tendency to keep his foot stationary and rigid when receiving a pass, and the ball rebounds too far from him. Or maybe Matt continually looks at the ball when he's dribbling, and doesn't see open teammates to pass to or defenders who are coming in to tackle the ball. Give Bobby and Matt brief instruction during the game, reminding them of the proper techniques they have been taught.

Games are for playing, not for detailed instruction. Your players' focus should be on the game. Save the more detailed instruction and technique practice for your next practice.

Player Substitutions

There are three issues to consider as you plan your player substitutions:

- Playing time
- Rotating players at various positions
- In-game substitutions

Playing Time

Is equal playing time appropriate? Is it fair? Should your less talented players play as much as your more talented players?

The first question to answer is actually this one: Does your league require equal playing time? Some leagues do, but some don't. Often, as the kids get older, this requirement—if in place at all—is dropped.

If it is in place, you need to have a plan that results in your players getting an equal amount of time.

If it's not in place, you need to decide whether you think an equal-playing-time policy is fitting. There are two camps of thought here. They go something like this:

- **For equal playing time**—"The outcome of the game isn't as important as it is for the players to develop their skills and have fun. How are the lesser-skilled players going to develop their skills if they don't play? And what's the fun of standing on the sidelines?"

- **Against equal playing time**—"Why punish the better players by taking them out, and why risk losing by playing your less skilled players as much as your more talented athletes? That's not teaching the kids realistic lessons about competition, anyway, because in all other aspects of life the emphasis is on winning and the attitude is dog-eat-dog."

Equal playing time makes sense, whether it's league policy or not, for players eight years old and younger. After that, playing time should shift more and more to the better players, though less skilled players should still get decent chunks of playing time at ages 9 and 10. By 11 and 12, most of the playing time normally goes to the better athletes.

Think through your substitution plan before you get to the field. You might want to work out, before your season begins, three separate plans, based on different numbers of players

note

In some leagues, you can substitute on-the-fly, as action is ongoing. In other leagues, you can only substitute when there's a break in the action. Check your league rules on when you can substitute.

showing up. For example, if you are assigned 12 players, make out substitution plans for 10, 11, and 12 players showing up. Bring each sample to the field with you, and then use whichever one applies for that game.

Rotating Players in Different Positions

Rotating players on and off the field is one issue; rotating players in different positions is another. The question here is, do you have players specialize at one or two positions, do you give every player relatively equal time in every position, or do you do something in between?

As with the equal playing time issue, there are different schools of thought on this subject. A couple of them go something like this:

- **Don't move players around in different positions**—"If Greg can't mark well at all, why put him on defense and make it evident to the whole world? And why embarrass him in doing so? Besides, kids won't develop their soccer skills at any one position if they keep getting bounced around. You're harming the players by doing this, not helping them."

- **Give players equal playing time at all positions**—"Youth soccer is all about learning the various positions and getting a feel for each one. Later kids can begin to specialize. Besides, the shifting around emphasizes the fact that, at this level, the game's focus is on learning, player development, and fun."

There is truth to each school of thought. Consider the following guidelines as you decide whether to rotate players and, if so, how often you should rotate them and to how many positions.

Players 6–9 Years Old

For ages 6–9, rotate players freely. This is their introduction to the sport, and there's no reason to pigeonhole kids at this point.

However, one caveat with that statement: If you have a child who is fearful of playing goalkeeper, don't play him there unless, through practice, he becomes comfortable at the position. There's no need to have every player play goalie.

When you rotate, choose one option or the other: either quarter by quarter or game by game. I've seen both situations work well, though I would use the quarter-by-quarter approach only for younger players and have a set strategy for player rotation there, as opposed to making it up on-the-fly every quarter. For example, your defenders could become midfielders after the first quarter and forwards after the second. Admittedly, it's easier rotating game by game.

Players 10+ Years Old

If you are coaching 10-year-olds or above, you might still rotate players some, but be more selective about your rotation, and it's good to settle on one or two positions for most players at this point. Why? They've had the opportunity to play in most or all of the positions, and it's time for them to begin to develop the skills that are specific to one or two positions.

Generally, place your stronger players in the middle of the field, and your weaker players on wide areas, and try to keep a balanced team, so you don't have all your strong players out there at once and all your weak players out there at another time. By and large, try to place your players in the positions where they will most excel and help the team.

In-game Substitutions

One of your game responsibilities is to make substitutions. At the earlier ages, make your substitutions to ensure all players get about equal playing time; this was already covered in the section "Playing Time." For ages 10 and above, here are some ideas for making substitutions:

- **When a player is especially tired**—Watch for players who are flagging. Get them off the field, give them a break, and put some fresh legs in there.

- **To gain an advantage**—If you see that by subbing in one of your players you will gain an advantage in a match-up, then do it, as long as you're being fair to the player who's being replaced on the field.

- **When a player is mismatched**—When you're on the short end of a mismatch, you can either change assignments within the players on the field or look to replace the mismatched player at an opportune time. But keep in mind the next item in this list; it's best not to take out a player after he has goofed up. If he's simply mismatched, though, and you have a better defender, make the switch.

- **When a player has done something good**—Surprised? I'm not suggesting you take out a player anytime she does something good; I'm saying when it's time to sub for her, look to take her out after she's made a good play, rather than a mistake. Taking her out after a mistake sends the message you're yanking her because she goofed up. Take her out after a good play, congratulate her, give her a breather, and put her back in a little later.

tip

Before you make a substitution, let the player who's going in know who she's going in for and who she's marking. Ideally, tell her this at least 1 minute before she goes in, so she can watch the player she's going to mark and get mentally prepared.

Appropriate Behavior

Remember that all eyes are upon you, at one time or another, during a game. Of most importance are the eyes of your players. They see how you behave, and that greatly impacts how they behave, or at least how they think they should behave.

Be positive, be encouraging, and cheer your team on. If you want to discuss a play with a referee, do so respectfully after the game. While you're on the field, respect his calls, make it clear to your players that you expect them to do the same, and punish or reprimand any of your players who do not respect the referee's decisions.

Coach your players to be good sports, and lead the way by being one yourself. Don't argue with opposing coaches, don't say derogatory things to opposing players, and don't root *against* the opposing team. Simply root *for* your team.

Coach your players to play hard, to play fair, and to play to win. Let your players know in advance how you will respond if they do or say something unsporting at a game, and follow through. For a mild infraction of your rules, talk to them, correct them, and give them one more chance. For a second mild infraction, take them out of the game. For a major infraction, even if it's the first, take them out of the game. In either case, consider suspending them for another game if you believe the infraction warrants such a response.

Sports offer an arena for kids to not only practice their physical skills, but also learn discipline, the proper expression of emotion, patience, and respect for themselves and others. And the person they learn most from is you.

After the Game

After the game, line your players up for a team handshake with their opponents. (Instruct your players in practice how you want them to behave during this post-game handshake.) Have them shake or slap hands and offer "Good game" or some similar comment to their opponents. Be clear with your players that you want them to refrain from saying anything derogatory, no matter what happened during the game. The team handshake is an important part of youth sports because it teaches respect for the opponent and helps keep the contest in perspective.

If you win, celebrate, but do so in a manner that doesn't rub it in to the other team. If you lose, don't hang your heads. Either way, go through the team handshake, thank the referees for taking their time to officiate, and then return to your side of the field for a brief post-game meeting.

Team Meeting

Hold a brief meeting before letting the kids go. This isn't the time to go into great detail, but let them know what they did well, what they still need to work on, and give them some positives to take home. Note areas where they have improved, note plays or situations in which they performed well, and help them keep the outcome in perspective. Help them learn from the game, whether they won or lost. For some thoughts on what you can learn from winning and losing, see the following sidebar, "Lessons of the Game."

Finally, remind your players of the next practice or game, and make sure they all have rides before you leave the field. Don't leave a child waiting for a ride, even if he says he's waiting to be picked up by a parent; make sure he gets his ride before you leave.

LESSONS OF THE GAME

What can players learn from a win? They can learn that

- Hard effort sometimes pays off. So, maybe all that time spent in practice is worth it after all!
- Sometimes you're better than the other team, and it shows. But don't rest on your laurels because another game is coming.
- Sometimes you get lucky. The best team doesn't always win, and your team can win on any given day.
- Winning is a team effort. Contributions to a win can come from unexpected places.

A win feels great, so celebrate. But remember the following:

- A win is good for only one game. Don't get too cocky.
- You don't have to be perfect to win. Don't get down on yourself for a few poor plays.
- A game's not over until the clock reads 0:00. Never give up.
- Soccer is a game in which you can redeem yourself. A great tackle or shot can erase that earlier error you made.

Soccer is a game through which players can learn about respect, hard work, teamwork, patience, persistence, and much more. It's also a game that teaches through defeat. Losses are never fun, but through a loss, players can learn the following:

- Sometimes you're better than the other team, and you still lose.
- Sometimes the other team is simply better than you.
- Sometimes you just have an off day, or you get unlucky.
- Sometimes you can work really hard and still lose.

Losing doesn't feel so hot. But remember the following:

- A loss is only for one game. Don't get too down.
- Pride comes before a fall. Don't chalk up a win before you take to the field.
- A game's not over until the clock reads 0:00. Never think you can coast home to victory.

THE ABSOLUTE MINIMUM

This chapter helped you consider all the issues involved in coaching during games. Among the key points were

- At the practice before the game, go over the game particulars—the field location, the time you want players to arrive, and so forth—and the game plan.

- Keep your tactics simple, especially at younger levels.

- Base your game plan and tactics on your team's strengths and abilities and on the opponent's weaknesses.

- Save the pregame speech. Just help your players focus on the fundamentals and game plan.

- Be aware of the signs of over-coaching and of under-coaching and steer toward a happy medium, being involved and encouraging but not directing your players' every move.

- Give your players guidance and technique tips, but don't overload them with information or corrections during games.

- Consider playing time issues and plan to give your players appropriate time on the field.

- At younger ages, move players around to various positions, but by age 10, have them start to hone their skills at one or two positions.

- Display appropriate behavior at games. Remember that you are your players' role model.

- Lead your team in post-game handshakes with the opponents and hold a brief meeting afterward. Help your players take home positives from the game, regardless of the outcome.

- Help your players learn from both wins and losses.

8

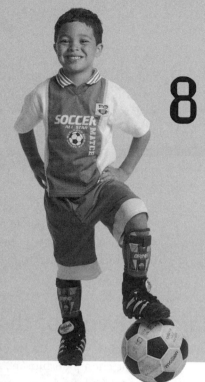

INGREDIENTS OF A SUCCESSFUL SEASON

The final game of the season is over and your players shake hands with the opponents. You hold a brief team meeting, and afterward, as most of the other team's players depart, many of your players hang around with their parents or friends, joking and having fun. A handful of players start an impromptu keep-away game. Four others race from one end of the field to the other to see who is fastest. You watch Chris, Dante, Kyle, and Megan sprint down the field, running off energy you wish you could bottle and store for yourself.

And you can't help but smile. "Hey, you goofballs!" you call out to the four speedsters. "Why didn't you run that fast during games?"

To a casual observer, it would be hard to tell that your team had just lost its final game, 7-3, finishing with a 4-8 record. That casual observer might think, from the way your team is carrying on, that you just won the league championship.

You didn't, at least numbers-wise. You finished in the lower half of the pack. But soccer is so much more than numbers. And, for that matter, success at the youth level is so much more than winning percentages, league titles, and trophies.

There's nothing wrong, of course, with winning the league title or having a good winning percentage. In fact, that's what every team strives for. Those just aren't the only indicators of success, and you need to measure your accomplishments as a coach in other ways.

Why? There are many answers to that question, but two will suffice here. First, the hand you were dealt, in terms of player talent, doesn't always come up aces. Sometimes it comes up a mixture of low, unmatched cards. Second, the winning percentage or league trophy simply doesn't tell the complete story. Consider the following two cases.

A Tale of Two Coaches

The Tigers compiled a 10-2 regular season record and went on to win the Border League championship. Yet, after the title game, the players' celebration was strangely subdued, showing as much relief as joy. Coach McReady didn't take part in the celebration, but watched it with an air of satisfaction and pride. No player came over to congratulate Coach McReady, and he made no move to congratulate any player.

At a players-only pizza party that night, the conversation went like this:

"I'm glad that's over."

"Me too. I couldn't wait."

"I wonder what Coach McReady would have said if we lost?"

"Probably what he said after our two regular season losses, only 10 times worse."

"I'm not playing next year."

"Me either."

"Why not?"

"Are you kidding? You want to go through that again?"

Coach McReady got the most out of his players' ability. He knew the game, he knew the skills and how to teach them, and he prepared his players to compete.

But he also trampled all over them emotionally and psychologically. Three players played the absolute minimum the league would allow. He yelled at players for making mistakes, the veins sticking out in his neck as he did, and he yanked kids out of the game for every error they made. He made them do pushups or run laps if their play wasn't up to his standards. He screamed at them when they missed a scoring opportunity or when they didn't immediately shut down their opponents' attack. He howled in apparent pain when the opponents scored a goal, no matter what the situation was. In his mind, the opponents should *never* score. He berated the referees; no one liked to referee the Tigers' games.

No one caught him smiling all season long. His normal pose was off to the side, scowling, his arms folded across his thick chest, a critical look in his eye. He shouted harshly enough at four players to make them cry, and when they cried, he ridiculed them for being babies.

The Jets, on the other hand, finished the regular season at 4-8 and got knocked out of the playoffs in the first round, losing 4-3 to the Tigers. (After that game, Coach McReady spent 10 minutes lambasting his players for almost getting beat by "a bunch of pansies" and told his players they might as well go home and play with their dolls if they couldn't play any better than that.)

The Jets were disappointed that they were beaten, but they had a festive pizza party afterward, and the players presented Coach Giles with a "Coach of the Year" plaque.

Coach of the Year for a 4-8 team? Though it was not an official league award, it well could have been. Consider these items:

- All of Coach Giles's players were as happy and excited about soccer at the end of the season as they were at the beginning.
- All his players improved their skills throughout the season.
- They also gained in their understanding of the game's tactics and rules.
- The Jets played hard every game, getting the most out of their abilities. They never gave up, and they didn't mope after losses.
- They pulled together as a team, rooting each other on, enjoying each other's successes, and encouraging each other after a failed attempt.
- The Jets *did* win an official league title—the sporting behavior award as "Best Sports."
- Everyone played, everyone improved, and everyone had fun.

Of course, many championship teams are coached very well and are successful not only in their win-loss record, but also in the ways the Jets were successful. That wasn't the case with the Tigers and Coach McReady, however.

Which coach would *you* rather be: Coach McReady or Coach Giles?

Evaluating Your Season

If winning isn't the only way to evaluate your success, what are the measures you should use? What are the keys to having a truly successful season? Throughout the rest of this chapter we focus on those keys. They shouldn't come as a surprise to you because they're a summation of everything you've learned in the first seven chapters.

These same keys provide the foundation for Appendix F, "Season Evaluation Form." After you read this chapter and complete your season, use Appendix F to evaluate your own season.

Did Your Players Have Fun?

As you'll recall from Chapter 1, "Your Coaching Approach," having fun is the main reason kids play soccer. That's an easy enough concept for most coaches to grasp before the season begins, but once the practices get underway, that concept can get lost amidst the more immediate and pressing goals and duties of a coach.

Can you win without having fun? Yes. But consider this: By the time kids reach age 13, their drop-out rate from sports is 75%. Some of that attrition is simply due to a lack of ability to compete at their age level anymore. Some of it is due to new interests that take up their time, such as music, art, or drama. But for the most part, players drop out of sports because

- They don't get enough playing time. Consistently when asked, kids respond they'd rather play for a losing team than sit on the bench for a winning team.

- They don't learn the skills they need to be competitive.

- They feel like failures (mainly because they haven't learned the skills). Their coaches don't reinforce their competence or help them see the positive aspects of their performance.

- They receive too much negative feedback from coaches.

- The sports environment is too negative; it's not enjoyable to go to practices or games.

- They stress out over winning because winning is overemphasized.

- Practices are poorly organized, tedious, and boring. Drills are repetitive, players are inactive, and the fun is drained out of the experience.

"Fun," then, doesn't mean telling jokes at practice, or goofing off, or trying to entertain your players. It means giving them playing time and building their skills so they'll feel competent when they have that playing time. It means reinforcing the skills they have and helping them focus on their positives, rather than dwelling on their negatives. It means giving them feedback but couching it in positive terms. It means making practices active, meaningful, and enjoyable, using a variety of games and drills that are game-like and that help them build their skills.

What are indications that your players are having fun? It's easy to see in the smiles on their faces, their body language, their focus, their effort, and their encouragement of each other.

Perhaps the greatest indication of all, though, is that they're happy at the end of the season, no matter what their record was and they can't wait for next soccer season to roll around.

Did Your Players Learn New Skills and Improve on Previously Learned Skills?

In considering player performances, all too often a season is judged on where the players ended, without regard to where they *began*. The true measure of success here is how much your players improved over the season. If they were good to begin with and ended up being good, without showing any real improvement, something went wrong. If they were poor to begin with and ended up being average, that's showing improvement.

Here are some of the mistakes coaches make in this area:

- They lack the teaching skills or technical know-how to help their players learn new skills or improve ones they've already learned.

- They are poor practice planners, meaning they squander their practice time or run ineffective drills.

- They push players to learn too quickly or present advanced skills and tactics too early.

- They don't present advanced skills and tactics as the players develop; they keep them at an elementary level and don't help them hone skills.

- They focus on their better players and offer little help to their lesser-skilled players.

The best coaches can work with kids of varying abilities and help them all progress. They don't ignore their lesser-skilled players, and they adjust their teaching plan according to the skill levels of the kids, always gently pushing for improvement.

To foster such improvement, first you need to be able to plan and conduct effective practices. You also need a critical eye to assess talent and needs, the teaching skills to instruct and reinforce your players on the correct techniques, plenty of patience because players seem to sometimes take one step forward and two steps backward in learning, and the ability to encourage and support your players as they continue their growth.

Every season is a building season, an opportunity for players to become better, build on their talent and success, and come back for an even better year next year because they have deepened and broadened their abilities.

> **note**
>
> There's joy as a coach in watching good players perform up to their capabilities. There's even greater joy in helping lesser-talented players pick up skills and perform beyond where they or anyone else thought they were capable of performing.

Did You Help Your Players Understand the Game and Its Rules?

Lots of games are decided by players' physical skills—by their abilities to dribble, pass, mark, tackle, and quell the opponent's attack.

And a lot of games are decided by players' abilities to apply the rules and execute the strategies: Alex is offside and a great opportunity for a goal is lost. Darnell centers the ball in front of his own goal and the opponents score an easy goal. Stacie doesn't realize that, as goalkeeper, she can move on a penalty shot and allows a shot to get past her that she could have easily stopped. The list could go on and on.

It's tempting to focus solely on teaching skills because that's such an obvious need. But players, especially at the youth level, need to also grasp the bigger picture of how to perform those skills and how to use their abilities within the rules to benefit their team.

When you build the teaching of rules and strategies in to your drills and practice games, you are one step ahead of most coaches—and one step closer to building a competitive, savvy squad that knows how to play the game and does the little things right. These little things can make the difference between winning and losing and between players enjoying the game and being confused or disappointed.

Did You Communicate Appropriately and Effectively?

Soccer fields across America are filled with coaches who know their stuff but don't know how to communicate it. Why? Because they think their ability to talk qualifies them as good communicators. (Of course, having read Chapter 3, "Communication Keys," you know this is far from the truth.)

Some of the signs of poor and ineffective communication include

- Players don't learn skills because the coach can't communicate clearly.
- Parents aren't kept informed and don't know how to pitch in and help.
- Players hang their heads or begin to miss practices because their coach yells at, degrades, or berates them.
- Players look bored or confused because their coach uses 100 words when 10 would suffice.
- Players don't listen to their coach because he doesn't speak with command or authority. This has nothing to do with volume or gruffness; it has everything to do with understanding, preparation, clarity, and delivery.
- Players aren't sure what to do in certain game situations because their coach hasn't told them.
- Players don't pay attention because their coach doesn't know how to get and hold their attention.

- Players appear wary and unsure because their coach said one thing but her body language said something different.

- Messages get lost, feelings get hurt, and sometimes tempers flare because the coach is too busy talking to listen to players or parents.

- Players, parents, and coaches become frustrated.

Your ability to communicate has significant impact on your overall coaching effectiveness. As you teach skills, do you clearly demonstrate them and use language your players can understand? As you correct mistakes and encourage players, what does your body language communicate, and is it in synch with your words? Do you *listen* to your players' comments and questions, and do you read and interpret their body language, as surely as they do yours?

Did you communicate with parents before the season, letting them know your philosophy and coaching approach, your expectations of the players, and what the players and parents could expect of you? Are you maintaining a healthy flow of communication with parents as the season progresses?

> **note**
>
> Do you maintain control of your emotions as you communicate? Note that this doesn't mean you don't *show* emotion; it means you *control* it.

Did You Provide for Your Players' Safety?

Providing for your players' safety doesn't mean no injuries happen on your watch. It means, ideally, that no *preventable* injuries happen and that whenever injuries *do* happen, you tend to them appropriately.

It's all in the planning and preparation. You plan for safety; you take the necessary precautions; and (when need be) you respond to the abrasion, bump, bruise, or twisted ankle when it occurs.

You are on your way to fulfilling your responsibilities here if you

- Are trained in CPR and first aid.

- Have a well-stocked first aid kit on hand at practices and games, and know how to use it.

- Make sure you know of any allergies or medical conditions of players, and know how to respond if the allergies or conditions flare up.

- Warn your players and their parents of the inherent risks of soccer.

- Check the practice and game fields for safety hazards and eliminate those hazards, if possible, before playing on the fields.

- Enforce player behavior rules that enhance player safety.

- Provide proper supervision throughout each practice.
- Offer proper skill instruction.
- Take a water break during practice.

Did You Plan and Conduct Effective Practices?

If you played youth sports, you undoubtedly attended a practice or two in which your coach was winging it. His "preparation" time was spent driving to the practice field, and the drills he chose seemed to have no real purpose to them, other than to bore you to tears. You didn't learn any new skills or refine the ones you had; you simply spent time—and poorly, at that.

Have you spent time planning your season and your practices? Are you effective in running your practices? Signs of effectiveness include

- Kids pay attention to you because you have a purpose to what you're doing.
- There is no down time while you're trying to figure out what to do next.
- Players are active and engaged at multiple stations that you run simultaneously; they aren't standing around waiting for a turn.
- You use games and drills that are designed to teach a specific skill or tactic you want your players to work on that day.
- Your players are learning new skills and refining ones they have.
- Your players are having fun in practice.

There's one more sign you're planning and conducting well: *you're* having fun, too. When you're prepared and your practices have a purpose to them, it's enjoyable for everyone involved.

Did Your Players Give Maximum Effort in Practices and Games?

You might wonder why this question would be part of evaluating your success. After all, motivation comes from within; you can't make your kids try harder.

This is true. But you can create an environment that increases the likelihood your players will give full effort. Conversely, you can create an environment that stifles motivation.

Obviously, you want to do the former and not the latter. Before detailing the type of environment that motivates kids, let's consider the type of environment that leaves them high and dry.

Some of the ways a coach can demotivate players include

- Yelling at them for mistakes and for their general quality of play
- Comparing a child to a better player

- Having kids wait in line to take their turn
- Not teaching players the skills they need
- Appearing to not care about their performances or about them as individuals
- Playing favorites, and paying little attention to lesser-talented children
- Not listening to them

Some coaches mistakenly believe yelling is the best motivator. Their players do become motivated to behave in a way that makes their coach stop yelling, which, it might be argued, is the coach's point. But if you yell at a kid to maintain better marking position, using an angry or irritated tone of voice, the child will often respond by becoming tense and anxious, which increases the likelihood that he'll make another mistake the next time he's marking.

Is it wrong to tell the player to maintain better position? Not at all. It's wrong to yell it at him, showing your anger or irritation.

So, how do you create an environment in which your players are motivated to do their best? You do so by

- Teaching players the skills they need
- Giving kids specific technique goals to work toward
- Giving specific, positive feedback as players work on their skills
- Encouraging kids, especially when they get down, and praising correct technique and effort
- Helping kids take home the positives of the practice or game
- Praising hustle, desire, and teamwork shown in practice and games
- Running efficient, purposeful practices in which players are active and engaged the whole time
- Valuing each child for his or her own abilities and personality
- Caring about the kids as players and as children
- Listening to players

tip

Want to show your players how much you value attitude and effort? Give a "To the Max" award or prize for maximum hustle and effort at each practice and game.

When you create an environment in which your players are motivated to learn and perform, you'll reap the rewards in practices and games.

Did Your Players Leave the Games on the Field?

League games can be highly emotional events. The players are performing in front of parents, other family members, and their peers. They want to play well. They want to win. They want to have fun.

Then an opponent scores on a shot that scoots right between their legs. They miss an open teammate who was in good position to take a shot. They get the ball taken from them. They get beaten on defense. The referee misses a foul. They are playing against a team that likes to trash talk. They mount a comeback, only to fall short by one goal.

Individual failures and team losses are not easy to take, but all players have to learn how to deal with personal and team setbacks. Losing happens. In fact, it happens once a game. Kids have widely divergent reactions to losing. Often, at younger ages, you can't tell which team won by the responses and behaviors of both teams immediately following the game. Sometimes, though, defeats can have an impact on kids, no matter what age they are.

Realize that while they take many cues from you, they also are heavily influenced by their parents' views on winning and losing and by the cultural stigma attached to losing. Some kids take losing very personally; some feel it marks them somehow; some feel they let their teammates down; some respond by being poor sports; others don't know how to master the emotions that come with disappointment.

Part of your duty is to help them master those emotions, keep the game in perspective, and leave it (whether it was a win or a loss) on the field. They can't erase a loss, and they can't carry forward a win. They start out 0-0 in their next game.

Talk to your team before the first game about keeping the wins and losses in perspective, and then watch for players who are too high after a win or too low after a loss. Help your players keep a level head if they win a big game or play exceptionally well, and help them look forward to the next game if they lose or play poorly.

Did *You* Leave the Games on the Field?

Jerry was coaxed to coach the Stingrays, his son Brandon's team, at the last minute. He went into the season with much trepidation because he had never coached before. But he found he liked it, and he had a good team that played well—"in spite of the coaching they get," Jerry wryly told his friends.

They won their first three games, including an upset against the Panthers, the league's best team from the previous year. The Panthers had most of their players back.

In the next game, though, the Stingrays lost to the Eagles, who weren't all that good. To his chagrin and surprise, Jerry didn't sleep very well that night. He couldn't believe he could lose sleep over a youth soccer game. But he did.

As the season went on, the Stingrays and the Panthers were running neck and neck for first place. They each accumulated three losses in the regular season, and Jerry took each loss harder than the previous loss.

"It's all right, Dad," Brandon told his dad on the way home after the Stingrays' second loss.

After the third loss, Brandon said nothing on the way home because his dad was too upset. "There's no way we should have lost to the Gazelles!" Jerry groused to no one in particular as he drove home. "That referee was ridiculous."

That might have been true, but what was *more* ridiculous was Jerry's response to the loss. He not only didn't leave the game on the field, but also took it home with him, slept with it, and got up the next morning and dragged it to work with him.

It's easy to get wrapped up in the wins and losses, to care so much about the kids and want them to win so badly that you let the game's outcome affect you more than it should. Care about the outcome, yes. By all means care about the kids. But do what you want them to do: Leave it on the field and come prepared to the next practice to go forward, leaving behind any baggage from the last game.

Did You Conduct Yourself Appropriately?

As you know, you're a role model for your players. How good a model you are is up to you. A few signs of a good role model include

- You communicate in positive ways with opposing coaches and players and with referees.
- You coach within the rules and have your players play within them.
- You maintain control of your emotions in practices and games while providing the coaching and support your players need.
- You keep the games in perspective and help your players do the same.

Remember this: Briefly losing your cool does not necessarily mean you failed as a role model. In fact, you can use such an instance to send a healthy message to your players. When you admit that you made a mistake and apologize for it, you set a positive example for the kids.

Did You Communicate Effectively with Parents and Involve Them in Positive Ways?

Some coaches put up with parents. Others look to placate them and hold them at bay. Still others do their best to ignore them, communicating with them as little as possible.

These coaches are missing the boat. At worst they are inviting trouble, and at the least they are overlooking a rich source of support and help.

Parents are your chief allies, and most parents want to help in some way, to make the sport experience as positive as possible for their son or daughter. Yes, there are parents who present problems to coaches, but these are in the minority.

You read in Chapter 3 about ways to communicate with and involve parents. If you have healthy communication and involvement throughout the season, it probably looks something like this:

- You have few or no misunderstandings with parents regarding your coaching philosophy.
- You delegate responsibilities, sharing the workload with a lot of parents—and making your program stronger in doing so.
- You aren't as stressed as you might be, had you not involved parents.
- You appropriately address the few misunderstandings or concerns parents have.

When you have a good communication flow with parents and involve them in your program, everyone benefits.

Did You Coach Appropriately During Games?

Some coaches don't make the distinction between coaching in practices and coaching at games, and their players suffer for it. In Chapter 7, "Game Time!" you learned of the perils of over-coaching and under-coaching and the keys of effective coaching during games.

So, what does effective coaching during games look like? You get high marks for game-day coaching if most of these statements apply to your game days:

- You keep your strategy simple and base it on your players' strengths and abilities and on your opponent's weaknesses.
- You help your players get mentally prepared for the game by focusing them on the fundamentals they need to execute and on the game plan.
- You provide tactical direction and guidance throughout the game.
- You are encouraging and supportive.
- You give technique tips and reminders, and let the kids play, saving the error correction for the next practice.
- You tend to the kids' needs during the game—emotional and psychological as well as mental and physical.
- You help players keep the game in proper perspective.
- You use a positive coaching approach.
- You effectively rotate players in and out.

- Your players conduct themselves well during and after the game, including the post-game handshake.

- You hold a brief post-game meeting, giving the kids some positives to take home, regardless of the outcome of the game.

Coach games in a manner that helps kids develop their skills, learn the game, compete well, and enjoy the experience. When you do that, you're assured of a winning season, no matter what your record is.

Did You Win with Class and Lose with Dignity?

Many players learn how to dribble, pass, mark, tackle, and defend the goal. Plenty of players enjoy good seasons, and numerous teams enjoy superlative winning records.

Unfortunately, not all those players and teams learn how to handle their successes. Puffed up with their own accomplishments, they taunt or trash talk the other team during the game and celebrate the victory after the game in a way that rubs the loss in to the other team.

Your coaching duties don't end with teaching your team how to execute and how to compete and win. It extends to teaching them how to handle victories and defeats.

Winning and losing are part of life, and the lessons the players can learn through soccer can help them deal with wins and losses in other arenas throughout their lives.

Here's what winning with class looks like:

- You and your players shake hands with the other team, offering them congratulations.

- You thank the referees for volunteering their time.

- Your team celebrates fully but in a way that shows respect for the other team.

And here's what losing with dignity looks like:

- Your players don't hang their heads, no matter how hard the loss was.

- You and your players congratulate the other team, looking them in the eye as you do.

- You thank the referees for volunteering their time.

- You hold a brief team meeting and help the players regroup and take home positives from the game.

note

Kids can give their all on the field, but they can't control the outcome of the game. When you help your players build character, they will know how to win with class and lose with dignity.

The ability to be gracious in victory and disappointed yet not defeated when you're on the short end of the score is all about character. You can help your players build character throughout the season, not only in games but in practices as well. Players can build character by having respect for themselves and others, by caring for others, by maintaining their integrity, and by following through on their responsibilities.

Did You Make the Experience Positive, Meaningful, and Fun for Your Players?

This is what it all boils down to: Was the experience positive for your players? Was it fun? Did it leave them wanting to come back for more? Championships or winning records don't mean much if the players can't wait for the season to end and half of them don't return the next year for a repeat performance.

Was the season meaningful to your players? Did they learn the skills and tactics, the game, and the rules? Did they learn about themselves, how they respond to challenges, how to win, and how to lose? Did they build character? For some telltale signs of a season that was positive, meaningful, and fun, see the following sidebar, "Signs of a Season Well Spent."

If your players show at the end of the season the same zest and enthusiasm that they showed at the beginning, you know you did well in this area. And you can look forward to welcoming them back next season.

SIGNS OF A SEASON WELL SPENT

Here are some signs of a memorable season. Hopefully, you will be able to identify with some of these signs when your season concludes:

- "Yeah, we were 5-7. We lost a couple of tough games, and we had a few games where we didn't play so well. But you know what? The kids improved over the season. They were really clicking and playing well at the end. And they had fun through it all." —*Coach Wilkens*

- "Cody was the worst player on our team at the beginning of the season. He didn't really want to get too involved at first. But he really blossomed. He gained confidence, and his skills improved dramatically from beginning to end. You should have seen the smile on his face when he started handling the ball better! I had lots of kids who played better, but I was happiest of all for Cody." —*Coach Yarborough*

- "I'd say, 'Molly, do you understand the offside rule?' and she'd say, 'Yes.' Then she'd find herself in an offside position without knowing why. I'd say, 'Molly, two defenders have to be between you and the goal before you can be involved in a play.' And she'd say, 'Okay.' And in a few minutes she'd be caught offside again. It took her half the season to get it. But she finally got it. I thought her teammates were going to lift her on their shoulders when she finally understood what offside meant!" —*Coach Mancini*

- "I just want to thank you for working so patiently with Andre. I know he gets distracted and he sometimes doesn't listen, or he forgets. Your patience made a big difference—and it showed in his play." —*Andre's mother*

- "I was really impressed with your practices; the team Jeremy was on last year wasn't run nearly so well. Jeremy learned so much more this year. Thanks, too, for letting me get involved. I really enjoyed helping you out." —*Jeremy's father*

- "Thanks for being a good role model for DeShawn. He's so competitive and he *hates* to lose. It's easy for his temper to get the best of him. The way you kept your cool during games really showed him something. Every time he wanted to blame a referee or complain about the other team, you focused his attention on his own performance. I think he really grew up this season. Thank you!" —*DeShawn's mother*

- "Hey, Coach, is there a fall league?" —*Your players*

THE ABSOLUTE MINIMUM

This chapter focused on the ingredients of a successful season. That success can be evidenced in a good win-loss record, but that just scratches the surface. Digging a little deeper, true success in a soccer season is evidenced by these signs:

- Your players learned the skills, tactics, and rules they needed to know to compete to the best of their abilities.

- Your players were mentally, emotionally, and physically ready to play each game.

- Your players improved their skills and understanding of the game over the season.

- Your players had fun at practices and games.

- Your players displayed good sporting behavior throughout the season.

- You communicated appropriately with everyone involved—players, parents, referees, and league administrators—and involved parents in your program.

- You planned and conducted practices effectively, keeping players actively engaged and presenting skills in a logical order.

- You taught skills and tactics effectively, showing and demonstrating how they should be performed and putting kids in game-like situations to practice the tactics and skills.

- Your players gave maximum effort in practices and games.

- You provided the coaching the kids needed during the games.

- You and your players gave each game your best and, win or lose, you all were able to leave the game on the field and keep the outcome in perspective.

- You taught your players to win with class and lose with dignity and guided them in doing so, leading by example.

PART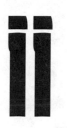

Skills and Tactics

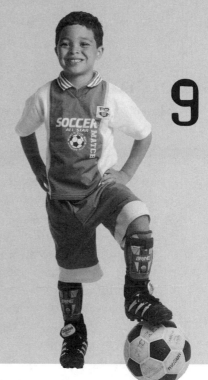

9

OFFENSIVE SKILLS AND TACTICS

In Chapter 5, "Practice Plans," you learned about planning your season and your individual practices, and in Chapter 6, "Player Development," you learned the method of teaching skills. Now, in the next two chapters, you'll be presented with the mechanics for all the skills and tactics you'll need to teach. Then, in Chapter 11, "Games and Drills," you'll find games and drills you can use to teach the skills and tactics.

In this chapter, the focus is on offensive skills and tactics—dribbling, passing, receiving, shooting, and so on. Use this chapter to learn about the proper execution of offensive skills and tactics and to refresh your memory before you teach the skills and tactics to your players.

Ball Control

You can't do much in soccer if you can't control the ball. Passes bound away from you, you lose control as you dribble, or your poor control skills result in you looking down at the ball and not seeing open teammates to pass to, if indeed you are able to retain possession.

Most players new to soccer think of playing the ball only with their feet. But as they'll find out, the ball will come to them in the air or on the bounce, and they'll need to learn how to play the ball with their thighs, chests, and other portions of their bodies—except for their hands and arms.

The best way to practice ball control is by juggling the ball. This gives players a feel for the ball. *Juggling* means keeping the ball going with your foot or thigh without letting it hit the ground (see Figure 9.1). This will be difficult for younger or lesser-skilled players, but they can start by

FIGURE 9.1

Juggling the ball.

letting the ball bounce once on the ground, then juggling it with their foot or thigh, then letting it hit the ground again, and alternating that way until they become more proficient at it. For more ideas on how to improve ball control, see Chapter 11.

Dribbling

The greater your players' ability to control the ball, the greater their ability to dribble it—that is, to control it as they move on the field. Dribbling is a skill that looks deceptively easy (at least when a skilled player is dribbling), but in reality it takes a lot of practice to master. Following are keys to effective dribbling.

Foot and Ball Position

Teach your players to dribble with the tops of their feet, contacting the ball with the lower parts of their laces (see Figure 9.2).

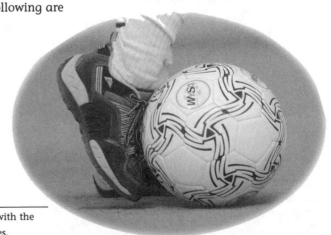

FIGURE 9.2

Contacting the ball with the lower part of the laces.

A common error young players make in dribbling is running with their toes pointed out, like a duck, so they can strike the ball with the insides of their feet. Instead, they should run with their toes pointed ahead, as normal, striking the ball with their feet turned slightly inward as they move forward (see Figure 9.3).

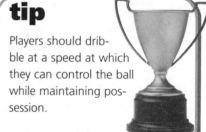

FIGURE 9.3
Striking the ball with the foot turned slightly in.

How far the ball should be from their bodies depends on how close defenders are. The closer the defender, the closer the ball should be to the dribbler's foot. If a dribbler is in the open, he can push it out farther from him to allow him to run faster (see Figure 9.4). He just needs to make sure he doesn't push the ball out so far that it can be stolen by a defender.

Inexperienced players often keep the ball too close to their feet, thus impeding their speed. Have players practice dribbling one-on-one against defenders to get a sense for how far they can and should keep the ball from them.

tip

Players should dribble at a speed at which they can control the ball while maintaining possession.

Players should practice dribbling with the inside (see Figure 9.5) and outside (see Figure 9.6) of their feet. This allows them to move the ball in different directions. They should also practice using their weaker foot as well as their dominant foot. However, it's more important to become adept at using the inside and outside of the foot than it is to become adept at using both feet, so don't overemphasize the ability to use both feet, especially at the younger levels.

FIGURE 9.4
Pushing the ball out farther in open field.

FIGURE 9.5
Using the inside
of the foot.

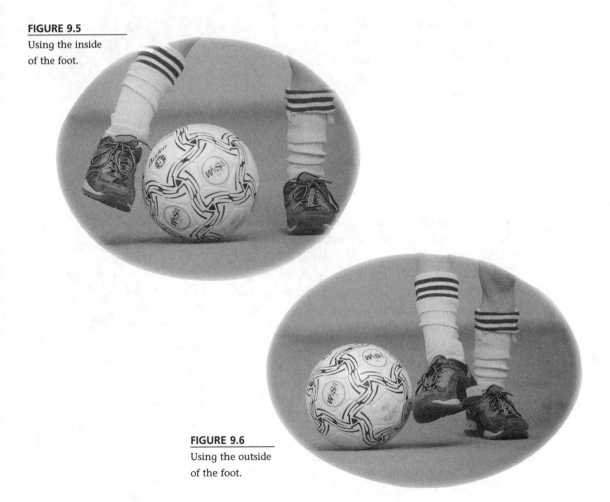

FIGURE 9.6
Using the outside
of the foot.

Head

There are two times when a player with the ball should have his eyes on the ball: when he first contacts the ball and when he last contacts it (that is, when he passes or shoots it). Other than that, he should have his head up, seeing the field, looking for open teammates and spaces, and watching for defenders (see Figure 9.7).

It's common for inexperienced players to watch the ball as they dribble. As they become more skilled at dribbling, they will become more at ease with looking up more often. And when they are able to keep their view on the field, and not the ball, they are much more dangerous.

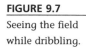

FIGURE 9.7
Seeing the field while dribbling.

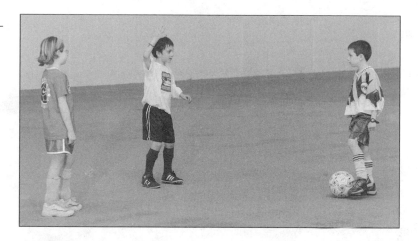

Shielding the Ball

One of the basic dribbling skills is keeping the ball shielded from the defender. The dribbler shields the ball by keeping his body between the ball and the defender. As the situation warrants—for example, when a defender is attempting a tackle or is closely marking—the dribbler turns sideways, shielding the ball from the defender (see Figure 9.8). Teach your players not to turn their backs on their defender; they need to be able to keep the defender in view.

Changing Direction

It's important for dribblers to be able to change direction because this ability makes them harder to defend. They should practice zig-zagging up the field while dribbling, going two or three steps to the left, then switching and going to the right, and so on.

The ability to use both feet comes into play here. The more a player is able to use both feet, the easier it will be for him to change directions.

Passing

A team that is skilled at passing is a joy to watch. Passing ability enables a team to control the ball, move it downfield, retain possession, and get open shots. Good passing is harder to defend than good dribbling because passes can go faster than players can run.

FIGURE 9.8
Shielding the ball.

Following are the techniques for passing with the inside of the foot, passing with the outside of the foot, and lofting the ball for longer passes.

Inside of the Foot

Passing with the inside of the foot is often called a *push pass*. Players use push passes for short or medium-length passes. To execute this pass, players should

- Lock their ankle,
- Turn their kicking foot sideways to the ball (see Figure 9.9a),
- Point the non-kicking foot in the direction the pass is intended to go, and
- Strike the ball below the ankle bone, close to the middle of the foot, contacting the middle of the ball and raising the knee up as the leg swings through (see Figure 9.9b).

(a)

(b)

FIGURE 9.9A AND B
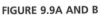
(a) Foot turned sideways to the ball for a push pass;
(b) contacting the ball.

Outside of the Foot

Players 10 years old and older should also be able to pass by using the outside of their foot. To do so, players should

- Lock their ankle,
- Bring the heel of the kicking foot behind the knee of the non-kicking foot (see Figure 9.10a),
- Turn their non-kicking foot slightly away from the ball to allow more space for the kicking foot to come through,
- Point their toe down and in (see Figure 9.10b), and
- Strike the center of the ball with their little toe (see Figure 9.10c).

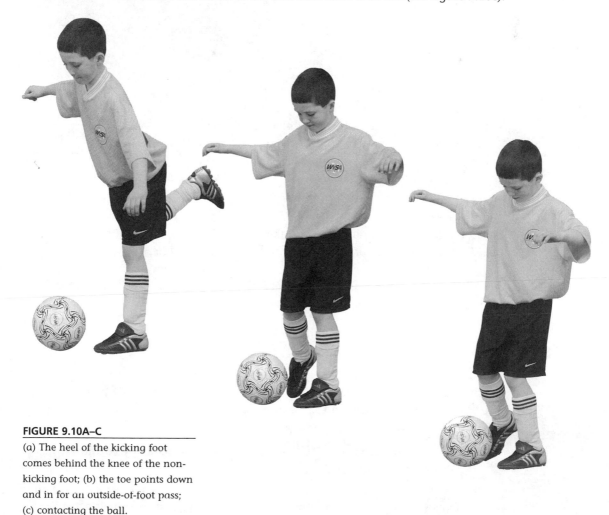

FIGURE 9.10A–C
(a) The heel of the kicking foot comes behind the knee of the non-kicking foot; (b) the toe points down and in for an outside-of-foot pass; (c) contacting the ball.

Longer Passes

For longer passes, players loft the ball in the air, using the top of their foot to do so (see Figure 9.11). The player plants his non-kicking foot slightly behind and to the side of the ball, points his toes down, and contacts the ball with the shoelace portion of his foot. By getting under the ball with the foot, players can loft it and get more distance.

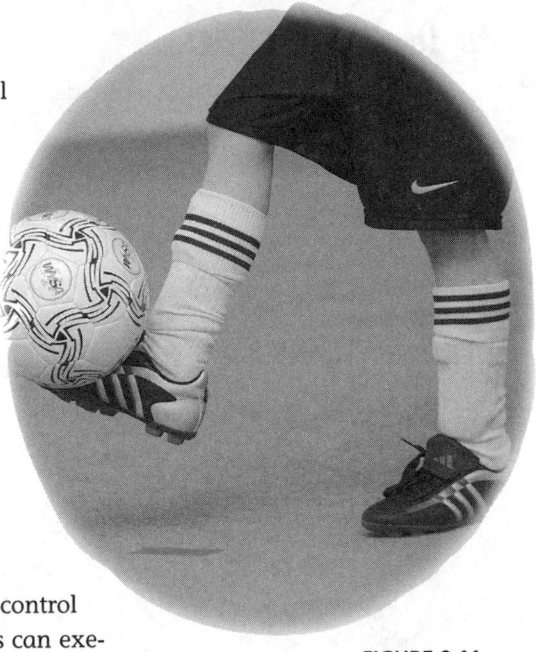

A Few Final Notes About Passing

A common mistake players make is attempting to pass before they have control of the ball. Sometimes skilled players can execute *one-touch passes*—that is, passes made on the first contact of the ball—but such passes are difficult to master. It's better to teach younger and lesser-skilled players two-touch passing, which involves a preparation touch in receiving the ball and putting it in a position to pass it, and the second touch in passing it.

FIGURE 9.11
Lofting a longer pass with the top of the foot.

Another common mistake involves the speed of the pass. As your players gain more control of their bodies and of the ball, they should become more aware of how speed affects the ability of the receiver to control the ball. Too hard of a pass and the ball rebounds far from the receiver; too soft and it is intercepted. As your players gain experience, they will get a better feel for proper pass speed. Guide them in this as they acquire and refine their passing skills.

Receiving

You can teach your players to be great passers, but if they don't learn how to receive passes, they won't get very far. Teams that are adept at receiving can control the ball, sustain an attack, and move into position to score.

When receiving passes, players should

- Read the ball, see where it's coming, and decide which body part to use to receive (foot, thigh, or chest).
- Watch the ball come in; draw back at the last moment, giving with the ball to cushion it; and control it with one touch, keeping it near their body.
- Look up to see the field after controlling the ball.

Players should have an idea of what they are going to do with the ball as they are preparing to receive it. After receiving the pass, they need to move their feet quickly to get into position to either pass or dribble.

Following are techniques for receiving with the foot, thigh, and chest.

Receiving with the Foot

It's ideal to receive with the foot because it takes one touch to control the ball, as opposed to two touches for any other body part (for example, a touch of the chest and then a touch of the foot to control it as the ball drops to the ground). Of course, the height of the pass has much to do with which body part a player uses to receive with.

Players can use their feet in several ways to receive. They can use the side of their foot to stop a ball in the air (see Figure 9.12a) or on the ground (see Figure 9.12b); and they can also use their instep to receive a ball in the air (see Figure 9.13).

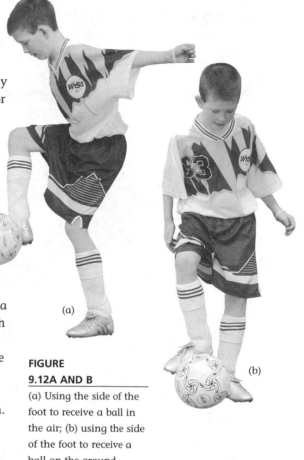

(a)

(b)

FIGURE 9.12A AND B

(a) Using the side of the foot to receive a ball in the air; (b) using the side of the foot to receive a ball on the ground.

tip

In receiving passes, you can't overemphasize the importance of giving with the ball and cushioning its impact to slow it down and control it.

FIGURE 9.13

Using the instep to receive a ball in the air.

Receiving with the Thigh

When a ball is coming in the air and is too difficult to receive with the foot, a player can use her thigh. To do so, she flexes the knee of the leg she is receiving with (see Figure 9.14a), cushions the ball by dropping her knee slightly just before contact (see Figure 9.14b), and controls the ball as it drops to the ground (see Figure 9.14c).

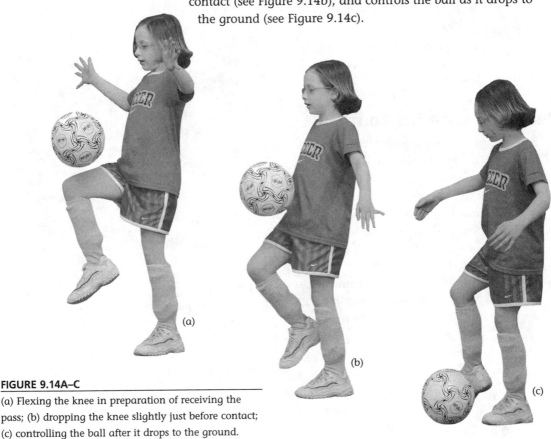

(a)

(b)

(c)

FIGURE 9.14A–C

(a) Flexing the knee in preparation of receiving the pass; (b) dropping the knee slightly just before contact; (c) controlling the ball after it drops to the ground.

Receiving with the Chest

When an airborne ball is coming in at chest level, a player can use his chest to receive the pass. The player stands in line with the ball's flight with his chest pushed out and his arms extended (see Figure 9.15a). Why is his chest pushed out? So he can give with the ball is it strikes his chest, pulling back to cushion the ball (see Figure 9.15b). As it drops to the ground, he controls it with his foot.

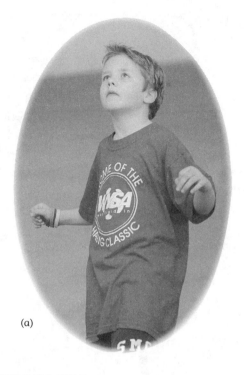

(a)

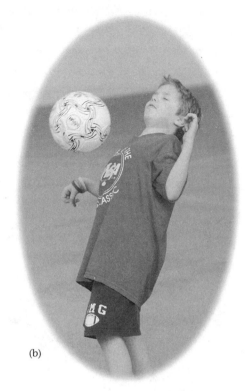

(b)

FIGURE 9.15A AND B

(a) Chest pushed out in preparing to receive the pass; (b) chest pulled back as the ball comes in, to cushion the ball.

Heading

Generally, when an airborne object is hurtling toward a child's head, we yell "Duck!" or "Watch out!" And the child's first instinct, regardless of what we yell, is to protect his head.

In soccer, of course, we want kids to forget what we've told them all those years about preserving their heads. In fact, we want them to use their heads not just to know how to respond in any given situation, but to receive passes or redirect the ball. Soccer is the only sport where "That's using your head!" can have a double meaning.

note

You should teach heading to players 8 years and older. Don't worry about teaching it to younger kids; they don't get the ball high enough off the ground to head it, anyway.

Heading the ball is not an easy skill to teach because of the fear factor involved. But if you begin gently, with kids practicing heading a ball that they toss in the air to themselves, they can become accustomed to the idea and can learn the proper technique.

To properly head a ball, a player should

- Keep his eyes wide open, his mouth shut, and his teeth clenched (this protects the tongue and tightens the neck muscles in preparing to hit the ball).

- Pull his head back and arch his back as the ball is coming in; his arms should be extended and his elbows flexed (see Figure 9.16a).

- Thrust forward and strike the ball with the center of his forehead, bending forward after contact to increase power (see Figure 9.16b).

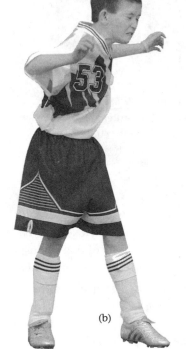

tip

Remind players that they are the aggressors in heading the ball. The ball doesn't hit them; they hit the ball.

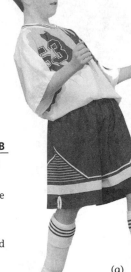
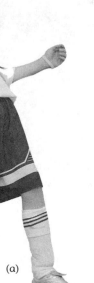

FIGURE 9.16A AND B
(a) Head pulled back and back arched in preparing to head the ball; (b) head thrust forward, using the center of the forehead to strike the ball.

(a)

(b)

Shooting

Kids love to shoot. But there's much more to the skill of shooting than just kicking the ball in the direction of the goal. When shooting, players should

- Approach the ball from a slight angle rather than from straight on.
- Take a slightly longer last step and plant their non-kicking foot by the ball with their knee slightly flexed (see Figure 9.17a). The non-kicking foot should be in line with the target. This longer step will help them draw back their kicking leg.
- Have the knee of their kicking leg even with the ball. If it's behind the ball, they have to reach for the ball. Doing so will cause the shot to fly too high in the air.
- Keep their head steady, with their eyes focused on the ball. Their shoulders and hips should be squared to the target.
- Strike the ball with their instep, with their kicking ankle locked (see Figure 9.17b).
- Drive through the center of the ball, following through for maximum power (see Figure 9.17c).

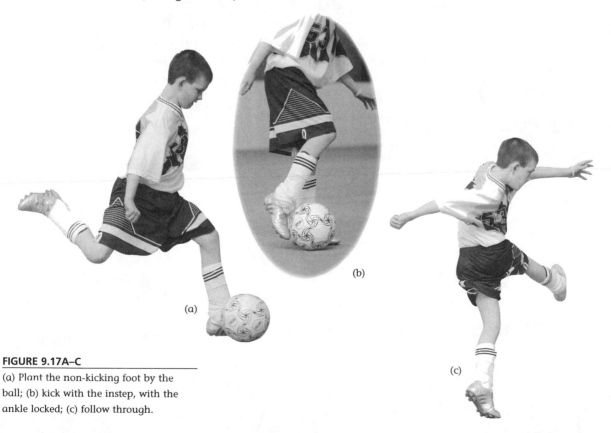

(a)

(b)

(c)

FIGURE 9.17A–C

(a) Plant the non-kicking foot by the ball; (b) kick with the instep, with the ankle locked; (c) follow through.

Formations

The positions of forward, midfielder, defender, and goalkeeper were described in Chapter 2, "Rules of the Game." Following are a few options for playing 6v6 (six players per team on the field), 8v8, and 11v11.

6v6

One formation you can try in a 6v6 game is a 2-1-2 formation (see Figure 9.18). In the 2-1-2 there are two defenders, one midfielder, and two forwards. In this formation, at least one of the defenders should help out on the attack.

Realize that younger kids will chase the ball like a flock of sheep all moving together. It will take repeated reminders from you to keep them in any formation.

A 2-2-1 formation (see Figure 9.19) presents a stronger defense because the 1 is the lone forward. Again, the midfielders need to push forward on the attack.

A 1-2-2 formation focuses more on the offensive end and is best run if you have a strong defender (see Figure 9.20). If your defender and goalkeeper aren't skilled players, it's probably better to stay away from this formation.

FIGURE 9.18
A 2-1-2
formation.

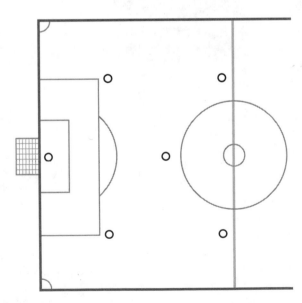

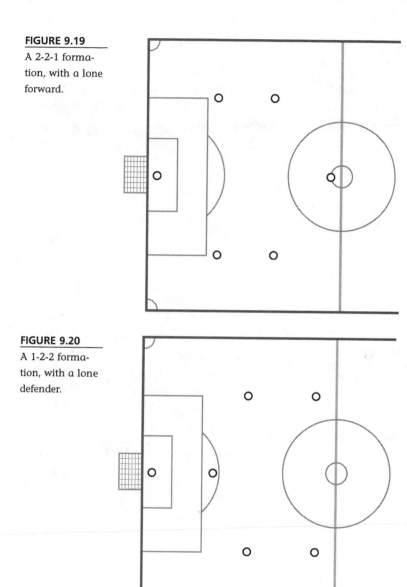

FIGURE 9.19
A 2-2-1 formation, with a lone forward.

FIGURE 9.20
A 1-2-2 formation, with a lone defender.

8v8 and 11v11

In 8v8, you might try a 3-3-1, a 2-3-2, a 2-2-3, or a 1-3-3 formation. Of course, the fewer players you have defending, the stronger those defenders should be. If you are facing a team with a strong attack, you would be wise to start with a 3-3-1 or a 2-3-2. If you're not so concerned with the opponents' attack—if you believe you have strong defenders who can manage well—then try a 2-2-3 or a 1-3-3 formation, placing more players at midfield and forward.

In 11v11 it's common to have four defenders, as in a 4-4-2 or a 4-3-3.

Support and Space

Inexperienced players often get a bad case of *ball swarm*. That is, they see the ball and swarm around it like bees buzzing around a lone flower. And why not? The object, as they understand it, is to get the ball and kick it in the goal. But swarming around the ball doesn't do much for your attack.

Instead of allowing your players to swarm around the ball, teach them these three important concepts:

- Providing support
- Creating good passing angles
- Passing the ball into open space

Let's take a brief look at each concept.

Providing Support

Rather than everyone in the same area code going after the ball, the nearest player goes for the ball and those near her fan out in support. In general, that support is best provided when the players form a loose triangle (see Figure 9.21).

> **note**
>
> Coach your players to look for open spaces on the field to move to when on offense to create pressure on the defense.

When your players spread out, it makes it harder on the defense because they have to spread out to cover their assignments. This also gives the player with the ball more room to operate, either to dribble or pass.

FIGURE 9.21

Providing support through the triangle concept.

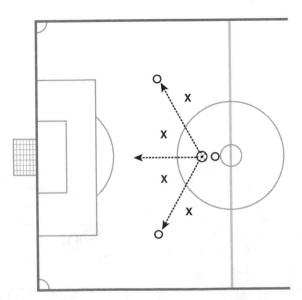

Creating Good Passing Angles

Teach your players to create good passing angles. The more options the player with the ball has, the more pressure on the defense. But if players are standing around and are not giving their teammate with the ball good passing lanes, they are helping out the defense.

Figure 9.22a shows a poor passing angle; Figure 9.23b shows the teammate moving into a position that creates a good passing angle.

FIGURE 9.22A AND B

(a) A poor passing angle; (b) moving into position to create a good passing angle.

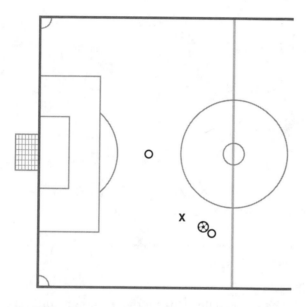

X – defense
O – offense
⊛ – ball

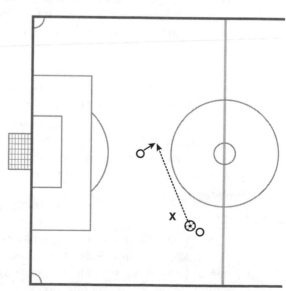

Passing the Ball into Open Space

The passer should pass to where her teammate is running to, not to where the teammate is at the time of the pass. If a teammate is breaking toward open space, the pass should go to that open space, timed so the teammate and the ball arrive at the same time (see Figure 9.23).

FIGURE 9.23

Leading a team-
mate into open
space with a
pass.

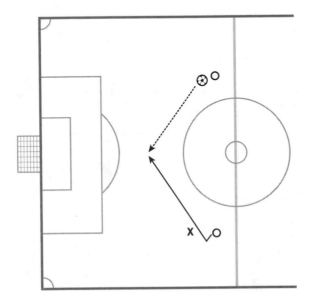

Attacking

The player with the ball should first look for the teammate farthest down the field (closest to the opponents' goal). If there's a passing lane to that teammate, the player with the ball should shoot a pass through. In this way, the ball passes many defenders at once.

If that option isn't available, the player with the ball should look to pass diagonally up the field. If this option isn't open, she should look to pass either to the side or to a teammate behind her.

Don't encourage your players to make risky or wild passes in hopes a teammate might get it. But do coach them to look for the best available opportunity. Above all, you want to maintain possession, and while you maintain possession, you want to put as much pressure on the defense as possible.

Crossing

Crossing the ball means playing it diagonally across the field from one side toward the middle (see Figure 9.24). This is done anywhere past midfield but is most dangerous to the defense if you cross while you're in the offensive third of the field, within striking distance of the goal.

FIGURE 9.24

FIGURE 9.24

Crossing the ball.

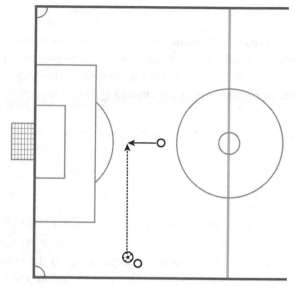

Give-and-Go

The *give-and-go* is a play that advances the ball past a defender. It is executed when the player with the ball gets his defender to commit to him, to mark him closely or attempt a tackle. As the defender makes this commitment, the player passes to a teammate and then sprints past his defender into open space to receive a return pass from his teammate (see Figure 9.25).

FIGURE 9.25

Getting the defender to commit and then passing and sprinting to open space to receive a return pass.

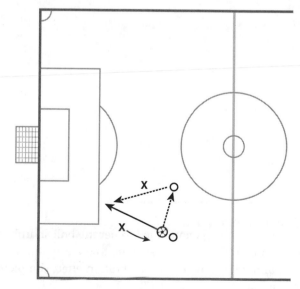

Throw-ins

When your team is awarded a throw-in, the player throwing in should immediately pick up the ball, hold it behind his head, and look for an open teammate. Generally, a throw-in should be directed up the sideline in the direction of the opponents' goal. Remind your players that they must keep their feet on the ground as they throw the ball in.

Instruct your players to move to get open for a throw-in, rather than standing around waiting for the ball to be thrown in.

Corner Kicks

A *corner kick* is taken from within the corner quadrant. The player taking the kick can't move the flag as she kicks.

The objective here is to get the ball into a danger zone. With the players positioned near the goal, the kick can be crossed across the goal for any of the three team-mates to play (see Figure 9.26). The kicker can shoot the ball close to the goal line, where teammates are stationed, or a little farther out, in the path of advancing teammates.

FIGURE 9.26

Placing a corner kick across the goal.

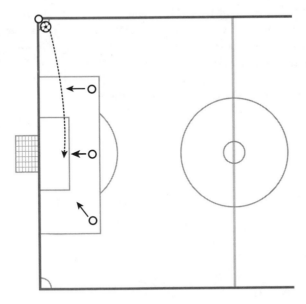

If the kicker doesn't have a strong enough leg to get the ball sharply across the goal, he can make a shorter kick near the sideline to a teammate who has a stronger leg. This teammate can then cross the ball, in effect completing the corner kick begun by his teammate (see Figure 9.27).

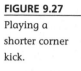

FIGURE 9.27

Playing a shorter corner kick.

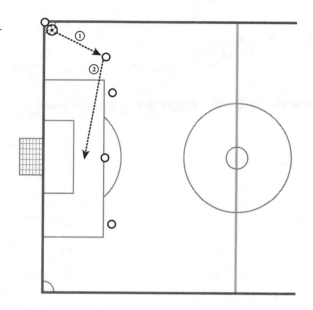

Goal Kicks

Normally, your goalkeeper will take your goal kicks, with the idea of maintaining possession foremost. One of your defenders should be on the edge of the penalty area ready to defend the goal in case the opponents regain possession.

The kick should never cross the ball over the penalty area; if the ball is stolen, the opponents are in a great position to score. Instead, the player could make a shorter pass to a teammate near a sideline or a longer pass up field.

Free Kicks

Always look at the referee to see whether it is a direct or an indirect free kick. A hand raised high in the air indicates an indirect free kick and requires the ball to be touched by another player before it can be shot in the goal.

When your team is awarded a free kick, the player making the kick should look to shoot, pass, or cross the ball, depending on her positioning and the defense she's facing. Often the defense will be aligned in a *wall*, with three or four players standing side-by-side; the player can try to shoot the ball through a gap in the wall, chip the ball over the wall, or pass to a teammate to begin play.

THE ABSOLUTE MINIMUM

This chapter covered the basic offensive skills of ball control; dribbling; passing; receiving; shooting; and various offensive tactics, including providing support and creating space, attacking principles, crossing, give-and-go, and more. Among the key points to remember are these:

- Ball control is one of the most important skills to learn. Practice juggling to acquire this fundamental skill.

- When dribbling, players should strike the ball with their feet turned slightly in, on the lower part of their laces. They should keep the ball close enough to maintain possession, but not so close to their bodies that they barely move.

- Passing is the most important skill. Players need to learn to pass with the insides and outsides of their feet and how to loft longer passes.

- They also need to learn how to receive passes with their feet, thighs, and chests, cushioning the ball so it remains near them so they can control it.

- When heading a ball, players need to keep their eyes open, keep their mouths closed, and thrust forward aggressively, striking the ball with their foreheads.

- A player taking a shot should plant his non-kicking foot by the ball and strike the ball with his instep. His kicking ankle should be locked.

- An attack is more effective when players provide support for the player with the ball by fanning out and creating good passing angles.

- Crossing the ball in the offensive third of the field is a good concept for players to learn because this puts the opponents in danger.

- Players making throw-ins should do so in the direction toward the opponents' goal.

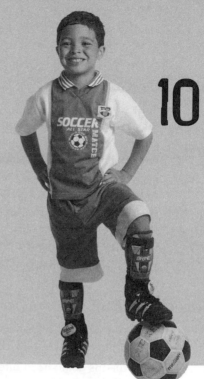

IN THIS CHAPTER

- Basic concepts
- Zone versus player-to-player
- Marking
- Tackling
- Goalkeeping
- Defending restarts

10

DEFENSIVE SKILLS AND TACTICS

In this chapter we present the basic defensive concepts you should teach your players and lay out the keys to executing the individual skills of marking, tackling, and goalkeeping. We'll also look at how to defend on various types of restarts.

In Chapter 11, "Games and Drills," you'll find some games and drills to help your players hone their defensive skills.

Basic Concepts

Players tend to be more tuned in to the basic offensive concepts—after all, most younger players enjoy the excitement of kicking the ball and their interest lags somewhat when the opponents have the ball. Remind your players that if they want to succeed and enjoy the excitement of attacking, shooting, and scoring, they have to learn to play good defense; otherwise, they'll not have the ball very often!

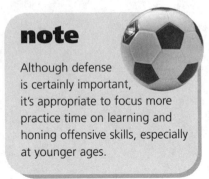

note

Although defense is certainly important, it's appropriate to focus more practice time on learning and honing offensive skills, especially at younger ages.

Following are some basic defensive concepts to teach your players.

Winning the Ball

Winning the ball is the most basic defensive concept. If you don't have the ball, you do everything you legally can do to get it, or win it.

That means going hard after every loose ball and looking for opportunities to win it. Teach your players to go aggressively after the ball, but to do so within the rules—meaning they should make sure that any contact is side-to-side or shoulder-to-shoulder; their elbows are kept in; and they play the ball, not the opponent. Any foot contact on the opponent is a foul.

Getting Behind the Ball

After the other team gains possession of the ball, the first thought in your players' minds should be: *Get behind the ball!* Teach them to retreat when the opponents gain possession. They should find the player they are marking or get in good position in the zone they are defending. The first instinct, though, should simply be to get behind the ball.

Jockeying to Buy Time

Jockeying the player with the ball means backing up a couple of yards from that player, keeping in front of her, and impeding her progress. This gives teammates time to retreat and get into good defensive position. This comes into play especially when the opponents first gain possession of the ball.

Protecting the Danger Zone

The *danger zone* is the area in front of the goal. This is where most goals are scored, and once the ball gets in the zone, your team is in greater risk of being scored upon. Your players should do all they can to keep the ball out of the zone. If it does enter the zone, they should do all they can to clear it downfield. One key here is to make sure they are never outnumbered in the danger zone.

The opponent with the ball should always be tightly marked in the danger zone. Even if your team is outnumbered in the danger zone, the nearest defender should take the player with the ball, marking him tightly to slow up the attack and hopefully to win the ball (see Figure 10.1).

FIGURE 10.1

Marking the player with the ball in the danger zone.

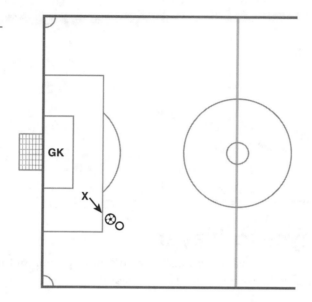

The Closer to the Goal, the Tighter the Marking

This is another simple concept: The closer the ball gets to your goal, the tighter your players should mark their opponents. In the danger zone, if the ball is close by, your players should be about an arm's length away from the player they are defending. If the ball is on the other side of the field, your players can drop off 10–12 feet (see Figure 10.2).

Closing Down the Attacker

To slow down an attack, the defender on the ball should close down the player with the ball. The primary goal here is to prevent the attacker from being able to turn and run freely with the ball.

Forwards Play Defense, Too!

When the opponents gain possession of the ball in your offensive third of the field, your forwards become defenders. At times, young forwards just stop after they lose the ball and allow the opponents to easily clear the ball to midfield. Your forwards are the first line of defense. If they can win the ball back, they are in prime attacking range. If they let the ball advance beyond them without playing defense, your team has to work hard to get the ball back to its offensive third of the field.

FIGURE 10.2
Marking distance
close to the goal.
Players on the
other side can
drop off a bit.

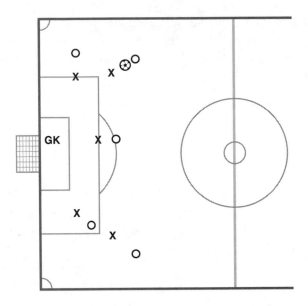

Zone Versus Player-to-Player

In a *zone* defense, each player is responsible for a certain portion of the field (see Figure 10.3 for a sample zone for an 11-player team).

FIGURE 10.3
Sample zone for
an 11-player
team.

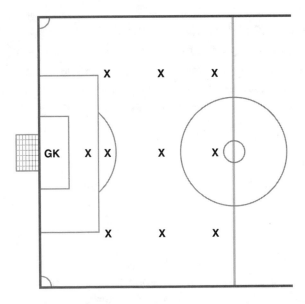

For 6v6 soccer, and perhaps for 8v8 as well, it might be easier to use *player-to-player* defense. Assign each player an opponent to mark. As soon as the ball goes over to the other team, your players should immediately look for the player they are marking and get in good defensive position.

Marking

There are several important concepts to teach in marking. One was already mentioned: The closer the ball is to the goal, the closer the defender should be to her opponent (that is, the tighter the marking). Another is to cut off the shooting angle if the opponent is anywhere near shooting range. A defender cuts off the shooting angle by making sure he is between his player and the goal, making it essentially impossible to score directly on a shot from that angle (see Figure 10.4a and b).

FIGURE 10.4A AND B

(a) The defender is not in good marking position because the shooting angle is open for the attacker; (b) the defender moves into good marking position, cutting off the shooting angle.

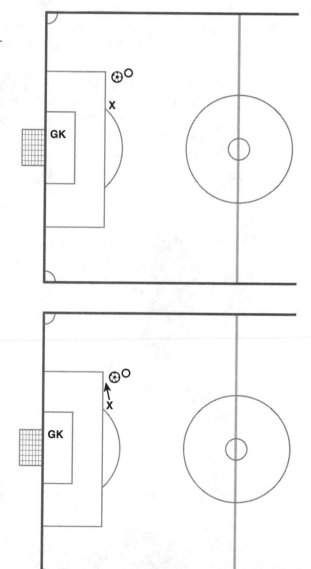

A third important concept is to always be *goal-side* on defense, meaning the defenders are always between their assigned players and the goal.

Keep your players focused on being goal-side, cutting off the shooting angle, and marking closer as the ball gets nearer to the goal, and they'll be on track to playing good defense.

Tackling

A defender *tackles* the ball by kicking or winning it away from an opponent. Players need to be aggressive in tackling, but they also need to be under control and not foul the opponent. They should kick only the ball, and not any part of the attacker.

The keys to tackling are good timing—knowing when to make the attempt and when the ball is most vulnerable—and control. Teach your players not to lunge recklessly at the ball, but to home in on it like a hawk on its prey, waiting for just the right instant to strike.

Players can use a *block tackle*, blocking the ball with their foot and driving the ball away from the opponent (see Figure 10.5a and b). Or they can try a *sliding tackle*, sliding on one leg and kicking the ball away (see Figure 10.6).

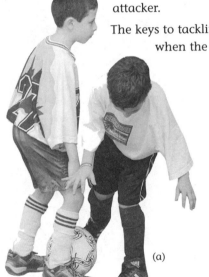

(a)

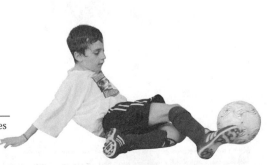

(b)

FIGURE 10.5A AND B

(a) A defender is in good position to make a block tackle; (b) the defender makes a block tackle.

FIGURE 10.6

The defender makes a sliding tackle.

Goalkeeping

It's good to have two or three players who like to play goalkeeper. Especially at the younger ages, interchange players at all positions, but if a few are more adept and more inclined to play in goal, let them do so. Just make sure you also give them opportunities to play other positions as well.

In the following sections, we look at basic goalkeeping concepts, on gathering ground balls and catching balls in the air, diving, and various ways to distribute the ball after stopping a shot.

tip

Don't feel the need to rotate every player to play goalkeeper. Play a few players there—the ones who want to play goal and who have good hands and the courage to stop shots. Confidence is a great attribute in goalkeepers. They should *want* to be tested by the opponents and be sure of their ability to stop shots.

Basic Concepts

Of course, the most basic concept in goalkeeping is stopping shots from going in. The techniques for doing so will be discussed in a moment, but first we'll focus on three concepts that are crucial to playing good defense as goalkeeper.

One of the most critical concepts of goalkeeping is to *narrow the angle of the shot*. The goalkeeper should do this at all times when the ball is on his side of the field, even if it doesn't appear that the opponents are in immediate position to shoot. The goalkeeper moves to give the attacker the least amount of goal to shoot for. Your goalkeeper can do this by moving forward in the goal, toward the ball (see Figure 10.7) or by moving to one side of the goal (see Figure 10.8). In Figure 10.7, the angle is lessened because the goalkeeper is closer to the shooter and thus presents a larger obstacle.

FIGURE 10.7

A goalkeeper advancing to narrow the angle.

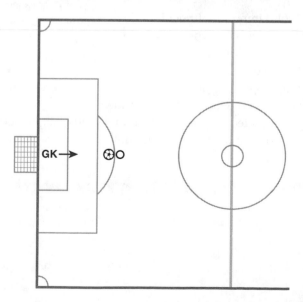

FIGURE 10.8

A goalkeeper moving to the side to narrow the angle.

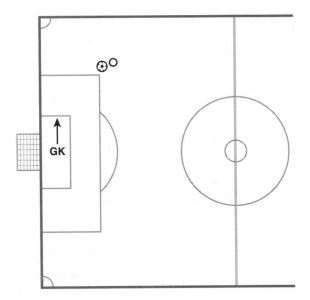

Another important concept is for the goalkeeper to get his whole body behind the ball. Sometimes, of course, this isn't possible, but the goalkeeper should strive to get as much of his body behind the ball as he can, no matter how hard or soft the shot is coming in. The more body that is between the ball and the goal, the less likely the ball is to slip by and go in.

Communication is also important in goalkeeping. The goalkeeper has the whole game in front of him. He should direct traffic; call loudly for the ball from a teammate so he can distribute it, when appropriate; and help teammates see and respond to threats and attacks. He should also let a teammate know if she is shielding his view of the ball. While a goalkeeper needs teammates to help him defend goal, he doesn't need them obstructing his view of the ball and the shot.

caution

When a goalkeeper advances to narrow the angle, he should be sure he can be in position to stop a shot before the shot is made. Also, he shouldn't advance so far that a shot can be chipped over him and into the goal.

Gathering Ground Balls

To gather a soft shot on the ground, the goalkeeper should bend at the waist and knees and scoop the ball with two hands (see Figure 10.9).

To defend against a hard shot on the ground, the goalkeeper bends at the waist; goes down on one knee, allowing no room between the knee and the opposite foot for the ball to slip through; and scoops the ball with two hands, with elbows tucked in (see Figure 10.10).

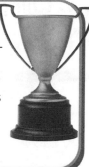

tip

Teach your goalkeepers to give with the ball, cushioning it by going back with it as they catch it, so the ball doesn't bounce away from them.

FIGURE 10.9
A goalkeeper scooping up a soft shot on the ground.

FIGURE 10.10
A goalkeeper goes down on one knee to scoop a hard shot on the ground.

Catching Balls in the Air

For shots that are coming in the air, the goalkeeper should do all she can to take the ball in the center of her body, gathering the ball to her chest and securing it with two hands (see Figure 10.11a and b).

For balls that come in chest-high or higher, the goalkeeper should shape her hands in the diamond position, with fingers spread and thumbs almost touching, and catch the ball on the fingertips (see Figure 10.12a and b). She should then secure the ball to her chest before distributing it.

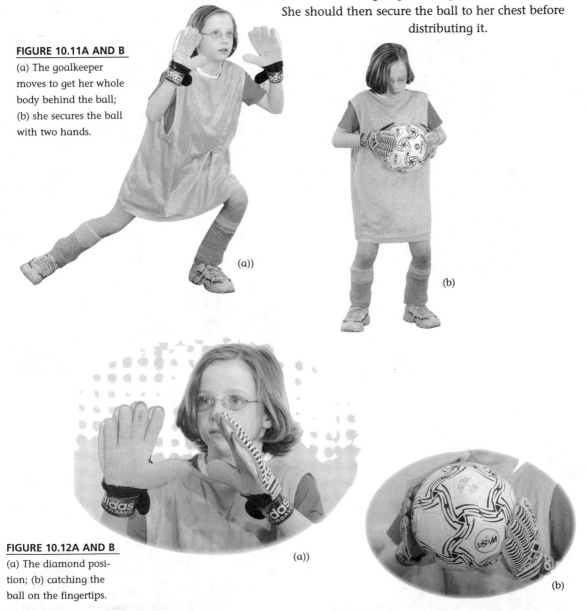

FIGURE 10.11A AND B
(a) The goalkeeper moves to get her whole body behind the ball; (b) she secures the ball with two hands.

(a))

(b)

FIGURE 10.12A AND B
(a) The diamond position; (b) catching the ball on the fingertips.

(a))

(b)

Diving

Instruct your goalkeeper to dive sideways, not belly down. Diving sideways will aid the goalkeeper in stopping a shot because his body will be turned to the ball, and it will also lessen any pain in landing (see Figure 10.13). His head should face the ball.

The ideal on a dive is to catch the ball. If the goalkeeper can catch the ball, he should secure it to his chest with both hands (see Figure 10.14). If it deflects off his hands, he should scramble to recover the ball before an opponent can reach it.

If he can't catch the ball, he should deflect the ball away from the goal, if possible. The main thing is to make sure the ball doesn't get past him for a goal.

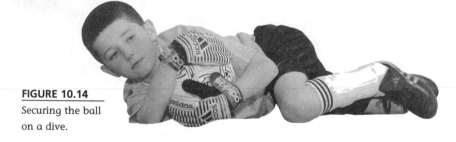

FIGURE 10.13
Diving to stop a shot.

FIGURE 10.14
Securing the ball on a dive.

Distributing the Ball

After the goalkeeper stops a shot, he starts the offense by distributing the ball. He can do this by rolling, throwing, or punting the ball. A goalkeeper cannot pick the ball back up after it has left his possession.

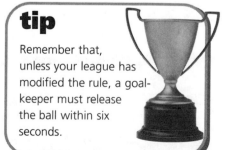

tip

Remember that, unless your league has modified the rule, a goalkeeper must release the ball within six seconds.

To *roll* the ball, the goalkeeper releases the ball at ground level so it doesn't bounce (see Figure 10.15). The keeper cups the ball in his hand, rolling it like a bowling ball toward his target.

To *throw* the ball, the goalkeeper uses an overhand or three-quarter motion, like throwing a football or baseball. The goalkeeper steps toward his target and throws (see Figure 10.16a and b).

FIGURE 10.15
Rolling the ball.

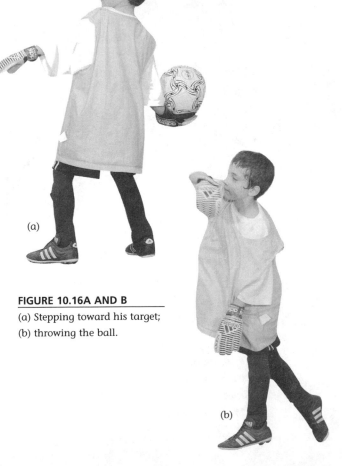

(a)

FIGURE 10.16A AND B
(a) Stepping toward his target;
(b) throwing the ball.

(b)

To *punt* the ball, the goalkeeper can either use a *full volley punt* or a *dropkick*. With a full volley punt, the goalkeeper holds the ball out from his body, steps forward with his non-kicking leg, drops the ball, and kicks the ball with his instep before the ball hits the ground (see Figure 10.17a and b). His feet and shoulders should be squared toward his target.

tip

Which way should your goalkeepers choose to distribute the ball? Have them roll the ball for distances of up to 10–15 yards, throw the ball for greater distances, and punt the ball to get the ball quickly into (or toward) the opponents' end of the field. Rolling and throwing are easier to control than punting, but punting can gain the greatest distance.

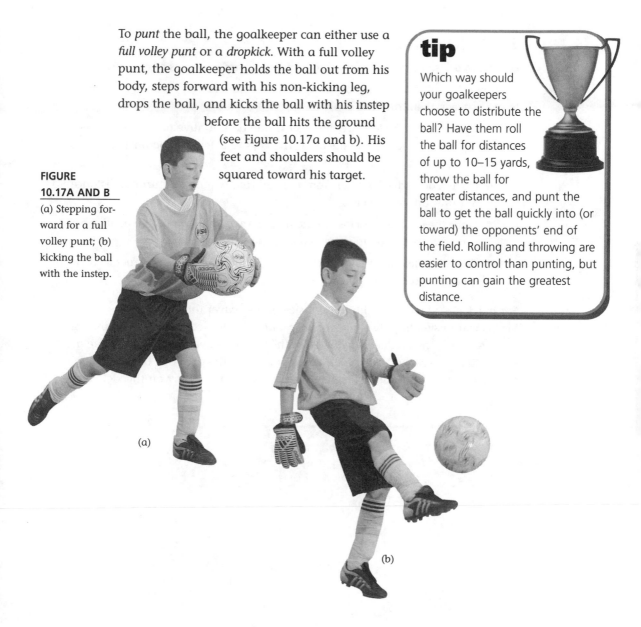

FIGURE 10.17A AND B

(a) Stepping forward for a full volley punt; (b) kicking the ball with the instep.

(a)

(b)

To dropkick, the goalkeeper drops the ball and kicks it immediately after it hits the ground. This type of kick is usually lower than a full volley punt and can be better controlled on a windy day.

Defending Restarts

Following are some considerations for defending various types of restarts.

For throw-ins, instruct your players to mark the players they've been assigned and to get between them and the goal.

Remember that corner kicks are direct kicks and do not have to be touched by any other player before going into the goal. The keys to defending against corner kicks include these:

- Place a defender 10 yards from the ball (the required minimum distance) to put pressure on the kicker.
- Place the goalkeeper close to the near corner of the goal. The goalkeeper should be prepared to move out or over to defend the goal.
- The other defenders should each mark their player, standing goal-side within a yard or so of their player.

For free kicks, players should get goal-side of the player they are marking. If the kick is within shooting distance, three or four defenders can form a wall that protects the goal. The goalkeeper can direct the wall to move left or right before the kick is taken. Between the wall and the goalkeeper, the goal can be covered on a free kick, making it difficult for the opponents to score directly off the kick (see Figure 10.18).

FIGURE 10.18

Forming a wall to defend during a free kick.

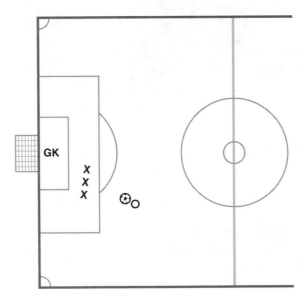

THE ABSOLUTE MINIMUM

This chapter explored defensive skills, including basic tactics and concepts, marking, tackling, goalkeeping, and defending during restarts. Among the key points were these:

- Basic defensive concepts include these: Win the ball. Get behind the ball. Jockey the player with the ball to buy time. Protect the danger zone. The closer to the goal, the tighter you should mark. Close down on the attacker to slow the attack. Forwards play defense, too.

- Defenders should remain goal-side (between the goal and the player they're marking) and cut off the shooting angle.

- Defenders can use a block tackle or a sliding tackle to gain possession of the ball.

- Tacklers should be aggressive but not reckless. They should go after the ball, not the player.

- Place kids at goalkeeper if they want to play there, have good hands, and aren't afraid to stop shots.

- Goalkeepers should narrow the shooting angle, get their whole bodies in front of the shot if possible, and communicate with teammates.

- Goalkeepers should gather ground balls with two hands, with their elbows tucked in, scooping the ball to their chest.

- Goalkeepers should catch shots in the air with two hands, giving with the ball to cushion it and securing it to their chest.

- Goalkeepers should dive when necessary to stop a shot. They should dive on their side—not on their stomach—and bring the ball to their chest after they stop it.

- Goalkeepers should distribute the ball by rolling it or throwing it to a teammate or by punting it farther downfield.

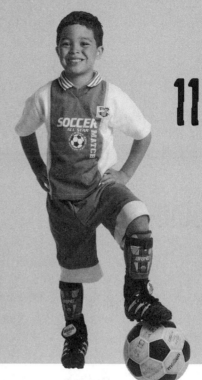

11

GAMES AND DRILLS

Now we get to what many coaches love: games and drills to use to help their players improve their abilities to execute the skills and tactics of soccer.

Use these 22 games as they are, adapt them to fit your needs, or use them to spur you on to creating your own games and drills. Know, too, that you can find many games elsewhere, including online. There is no lack of games out there. The challenge is to use games and drills that will benefit your players the most. Many games are boring, or make kids stand in line for a long time, or aren't realistic in terms of requiring kids to practice skills they will use in real contests. Steer clear of those types of games.

Instead, use games that put your players in game-like situations, that are fun, that call on them to execute the skills and tactics they will need to perform in real games, and that keep them active and not standing around waiting a long time for their turn.

Good luck in your season. Enjoy it, and help your players enjoy the great sport of soccer!

Dribbling Games

Here are three games to use to practice dribbling. Realize that most kids will dribble the ball with their toes or the inside of the foot and will have a difficult time changing direction. Remember to teach the proper form, dribbling with the laces of the shoe or the outside of the foot.

Game One

Name	Green Light, Red Light
Purpose	To develop dribbling and ball control skills. Players will keep the ball close to them and be able to stop on command.
Setup	Each player has a ball and lines up at one end of the field (see Figure 11.1). The coach is at the other end.
Description	When the coach yells "Green light," the players dribble as fast as they can until the coach yells "Red light." On this command, each player stops and puts a foot on the ball. If a player cannot stop and control the ball, she must return to the start. Repeat calling "Green light; red light," until someone wins the race by reaching the coach.
Notes	At first, some players will run out of control and others will walk, but you will see an improvement in both after a few weeks.
	A variation of this game is "Simon Says," in which the coach calls out "Simon says go!" and "Simon says stop!" At times, the coach can shout "Go!" or "Stop!" without saying "Simon says," and players who don't obey those commands must return to the beginning.

FIGURE 11.1

Setup for Green
Light, Red Light.

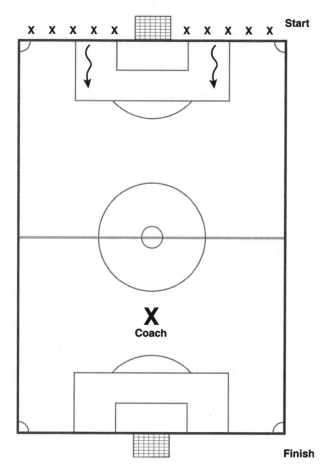

Game Two

Name	Sharks and Minnows
Purpose	For players to learn to dribble across an area while other players attempt to take the ball from them.
Setup	Use the length of the field for U-8 and under, and a 20-yard × 30-yard grid for older players. The Minnows line up at one end, each Minnow with a ball, and the Shark lines up halfway down the grid (see Figure 11.2). There is only one Shark to begin with.
Description	On the coach's command, the Minnows dribble as fast as they can, while under control, to the other end of the grid, as the Shark attempts to kick the ball out of the "sea." The Minnows who lose possession become Sharks. This is

repeated until there is only one Minnow left standing. He becomes the Shark for the next time.

Notes A variation could be that, when the Shark eats a Minnow, he becomes a Minnow and the Minnow becomes a Shark.

FIGURE 11.2

Setup for Sharks and Minnows.

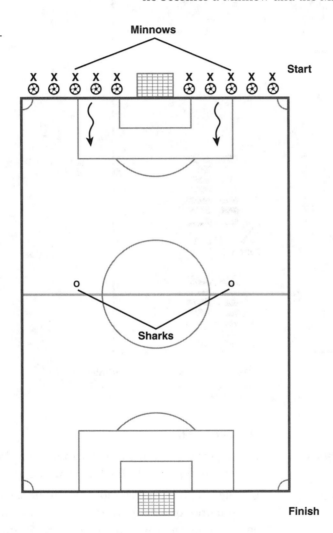

Game Three

Name Dribble Relay

Purpose To learn to use the inside and outside of the foot to change direction while dribbling.

Setup Divide your players into two teams of evenly-matched players. Using cones, set up an obstacle course for each team. Set up four gates about 10 yards diagonally apart.

Description The first player on each team dribbles through the obstacle course, turning right at the first gate, left at the second, doing a 360 around the third, a 180 at the fourth, and returning to the starting line, where she tags her teammate, who repeats the course (see Figure 11.3). Continue this until all players get to the finish line.

Notes To vary this game, have parents stand by the gates and randomly hold up a number of fingers. Give players a time bonus for calling out the right number. This will motivate players to keep their heads up.

This variation is better with players 8 and older. This is a great game to use to help players practice dribbling with their heads up.

FIGURE 11.3

Execution of Dribble Relay.

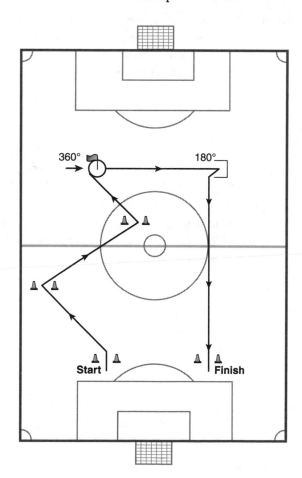

Passing Games

Here are three games to help your players hone their passing skills. Passing is the skill used the most in soccer. In a 90-minute game, a ball is passed 900–1,000 times! Passing is mainly about accuracy and pace. You should teach your players the push pass, chip pass, and long-ball pass.

Game One

Name	Monkey in the Middle
Purpose	To make push passes to teammates while keeping the ball away from the player in the middle.
Setup	A grid from 10 yards × 10 yards up to a grid 20 yards × 20 yards.
Description	Play 3 on 1 in a smaller grid to begin, and advance in later practices to 5 on 2 in a bigger grid. The player or players in the middle try to take the ball away from the other players, who move around in the grid and pass to each other (see Figure 11.4). Emphasize 5- to 6-yard push passes.
	When the ball is stolen by a monkey in the middle, the player who made the pass switches places with the "monkey."
	As players improve, set a goal of 10, 15, or 20 passes before they lose possession.
Notes	It is difficult to get 6-year-olds to pass the ball because they feel like they just got it. And often when they do pass, they toe poke it. Encourage them to pass it with the inside of their foot.
	Even with the older kids, it can be a challenge getting them to pass the ball unless they know it will be passed back to them. This game emphasizes looking for open teammates and passing to them—and receiving passes in return.

FIGURE 11.4

Execution of
Monkey in the
Middle.

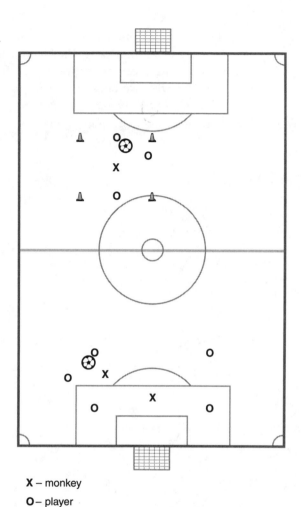

X – monkey

O – player

Game Two

Name	Pass and Move
Purpose	To get kids to move after they make a pass, rather than stopping and admiring their pass.
Setup	Have the players line up in three lines 10–15 yards apart starting at the goal line (see Figure 11.5).
Description	The players do a three-player weave up the field. It starts with Player B passing the ball to Player A. Player A passes to Player C and runs diagonally across the field while Player B runs behind and around Player A. Player C passes the ball to Player B and then runs around Player A as he prepares to receive a pass from Player A.

When players get good at this, you can toss in another ball. |

Notes　Several things are accomplished besides getting players used to moving after they pass. They learn each other's names; they learn to communicate with each other; and, when you play with two balls, they learn to avoid the other players. At first, the players will have problems getting the hang of the weave, but when they do, it will be very effective in getting them to move after passing.

FIGURE 11.5

Setup for Pass and Move.

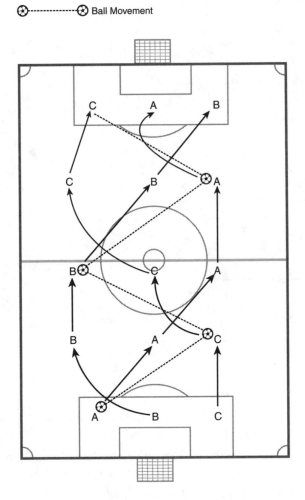

⊗------------⊗ Ball Movement

Game Three

Name　Soccer Golf

Purpose　Develops the ability to chip the ball 10, 20, 30 yards, and further.

Setup   Set up five tee boxes marked by cones and targets marked by flags (see Figure 11.6). Start a player at each hole.

Description   Players chip the ball from the tee box to a flag at least 10 yards away. If they fail to hit the flag, they must kick the ball again. Each time they kick the ball is a stroke; the player with the fewest strokes at the end of five holes wins.

          As players get better at this game, put obstacles (such as small benches or goals) on the course that they must avoid.

Notes   You can also make teams of two where players can alternate shots and one teammate can trap the ball or redirect it to the hole with no penalty.

FIGURE 11.6

Setup for Soccer Golf.

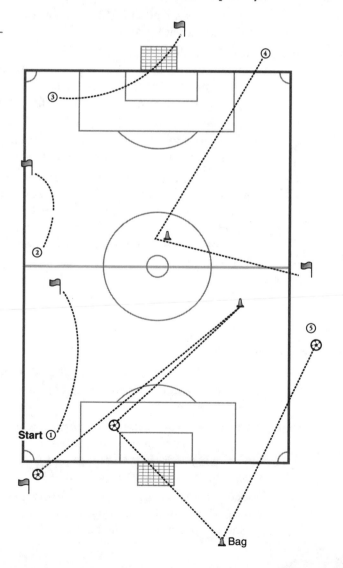

Receiving Games

The following three games will help your players develop their abilities to receive passes. Receiving can be difficult to master because it's hard to learn to cushion the ball so it stops. Encourage your players to trap the ball with the insides of their feet when it comes to them on the ground and with their laces, thighs, or chests when it comes to them in the air.

Game One

Name	Juggle, Uggle, Oops!
Purpose	To improve ball control, concentration, and touch.
Setup	Have players spread out with plenty of space around each one. Each player has a ball.
Description	Give players 30–90 seconds to juggle the ball with their head, shoulders, thighs, and feet. They get one point for each contact they make before the ball hits the ground. Then they start again, trying to beat their previous score.
Notes	At first, players might be able to do only one touch before the ball hits the ground, and that's okay. Encourage them to improve their score by one or two a week.
	They can practice this easily at home, and as they improve, they'll gain confidence and desire to improve other aspects of their game. Many kids will find this game frustrating and be embarrassed to do it in front of their teammates, so you might consider making this part of their homework.

Game Two

Name	Pop and Stop
Purpose	To develop the ability to stop and control a hard pass.
Setup	Have two lines of players standing 10 yards apart. Each player in one line begins with a ball and is paired up with a partner in the other line.
Description	Each player pops a pass to her partner, who has to stop it dead or at least within one step from his foot, using the inside of his foot. He then pops a pass back to his partner and the process continues (see Figure 11.7).
	Make sure the passing is not wild; the emphasis is on accuracy and control. Instruct your players to make their first 5 passes at 50% strength, the next 5 at 75%, and the last 10

at 100%. If you want, you can score the partners, with each pass that is not more than a step away from the receiver scored as one point. The highest score wins.

Notes When players get good at this, they should receive the pass in a two-touch motion, the first touch receiving the ball and the second touch passing it back. If players don't receive the pass correctly, they will not be able to pass it back with their second touch.

FIGURE 11.7

Execution of Pop and Stop.

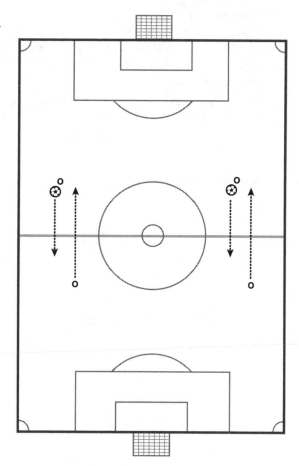

Game Three

Name Toss and Trap/Soccer Volleyball

Purpose To learn to receive a ball with the head, chest, thigh, or foot.

Setup Have two lines of partners face each other, 5 yards apart, on a grid 10 yards × 10 yards or 20 yards × 20 yards (see Figure 11.8).

Description   One player tosses the ball underhanded to his partner, who traps the ball with the appropriate body part—head, chest, thigh, or foot—and then passes it back to his teammate. The players repeat this 12 times, with the tosser making different tosses so his partner has to attempt different types of receptions. After the 12th toss, the tosser and the trapper swap duties.

You can convert Toss and Trap into a game of Soccer Volleyball by placing two even teams on each side of a line marked with flags (see Figure 11.9). To start the game, one team punts the ball to the other, and that team has three touches on the ball before they must return the ball to the opposing team. Allow the ball to touch the ground once per possession.

Notes   In Toss and Trap, it is important that the player tossing the ball does so in control and accurately, so his teammate can practice various types of receptions.

FIGURE 11.8

Setup for Toss and Trap.

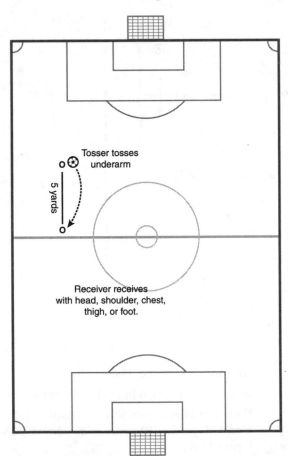

Tosser tosses underarm

5 yards

Receiver receives with head, shoulder, chest, thigh, or foot.

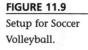

FIGURE 11.9

Setup for Soccer
Volleyball.

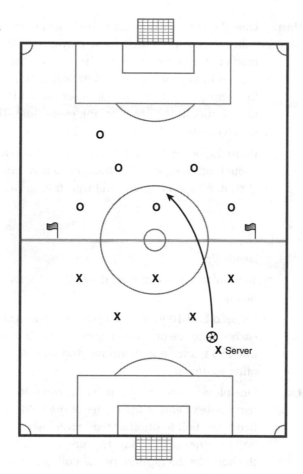

Heading Games

Here are two heading games for you to use. Heading is the art of redirecting the ball,
and it doesn't hurt when it's done correctly. But most kids have a fear of heading the
ball. Emphasize proper form, focusing on striking the ball with the forehead, and
eventually (hopefully soon!) your players will be able to use this skill as an effective
weapon.

Game One

Name	Head and Catch
Purpose	To develop quick and accurate response to ball movement.
Setup	Players line up in pairs, 2–3 yards apart from each other. Each pair has a ball.

Description   One player tosses the ball to her partner and calls out either "Head" or "Catch." The player receiving the ball reacts to the command and either heads the ball or catches it. Repeat the process rapidly for 2 minutes, with the same player tossing. The tosser should toss the ball underhand, at the same height, every time. The tosser and the receiver switch duties every 2 minutes.

Notes   Up to the age of 8, most kids can't get the ball high enough off the ground to head it, so if you are a coach of U-8s, don't spend much time with this game.

Game Two

Name   Heads Up!

Purpose   To maintain possession of the ball and score with their heads.

Setup   Set up a grid 10 yards × 10 yards with 1-yard goals on each side of the grid (see Figure 11.10). Divide the players into two teams, one group playing north/south and the other east/west.

Description   One player starts the game by throwing the ball to a teammate's head in the center of the field. The teammate heads the ball to another teammate, who can head the ball in either of the goals to score. After a team has scored, the ball hits the ground, or the ball goes out of bounds, the other team gets possession. A team cannot score in the same goal consecutively.

Notes   If players are struggling with keeping the ball in the air, allow them to use their feet every other time.

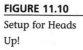

FIGURE 11.10

Setup for Heads
Up!

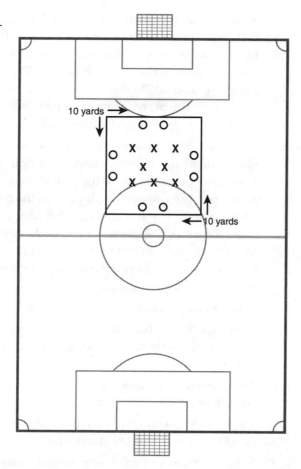

Shooting Games

The following three games will help develop shooting skills. Of course, kids love to practice shooting because they want the glory of scoring goals. These games will improve their chances of shooting accurately.

Game One

Name	Circle and Shoot
Purpose	To help players understand where the best places are to shoot the ball.

Setup

Set up a goal, preferably with no net. Each player has a ball. Place a cone in the middle of the goal, three cones on the goal line next to the left side of the goal, and two cones on the goal line on the right side. The object is for players to shoot at the three cones on the bottom-left side of the goal. The players start in one line but quickly spread out as they start shooting (see Figure 11.11).

Description

Players line up 5 yards to the left of the penalty box. The players take turns dribbling toward the right corner flag. When they get to the top of the penalty box, they shoot. Award points for where the player shot the ball. If the player shot the ball in the bottom-left corner and knocked down the cones, she gets three points. Award two points for shots in the lower-right corner or upper-left corner. Give one point for shots outside the post on the left side.

Players receive no points for missing the goal to the right or if the ball goes over the goal.

After shooting the ball, the player circles around the goal and picks up the ball, gets back in line, and repeats the process.

After three or four times going to the right, have players go to their left and shoot with their left foot.

Notes

When players get good at this drill, have your goalkeeper stand in the goal to make it more challenging.

To make this more challenging, deduct a point every time a player shoots over the goal or outside to the right.

FIGURE 11.11
Setup and execution for Circle and Shoot.

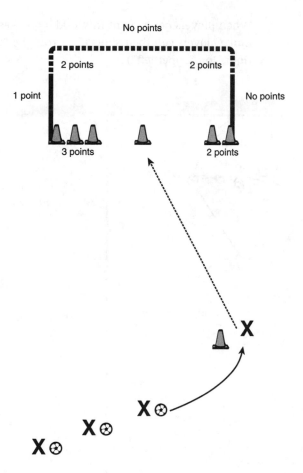

Game Two

Name	Run and Gun
Purpose	To learn to pass, run, receive a return pass, and shoot.
Setup	Place a cone at the half line and cones in the goal. Players line up in the center circle.
Description	A player passes the ball to the coach standing at the top of the penalty area (see Figure 11.12). The player runs as fast as he can toward the right corner flag, and the coach passes the ball to him. The player times his run to meet the ball and shoot it in stride. The player can shoot low or chip the ball. Repeat this process on the left side.

Notes   When players get good at this, add a goalkeeper and
make players call their shots (for example, "Chip," "Lower
right," or "Upper left").

FIGURE 11.12

Execution of
Run and Gun.

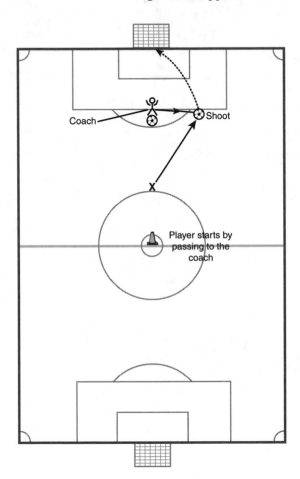

Game Three

Name   Kentucky Derby

Purpose   To run, shoot, and get back on defense. This game builds
endurance, shooting skills, and reaction time.

Setup   Set up two goals 30–40 yards apart with flags or cones
marking the halfway line. Divide the players into two
teams and line them up on the right side of each goal (see
Figure 11.13). Each team has a ball.

Description   Have a player stand in the goal on one side. At your command, the first player on the other side dribbles to the halfway marker and shoots at the opponent's goal. She then runs back to her goal and becomes goalkeeper for the opponent's first shot. After she has taken her shot, the player with the ball on the other team can start dribbling to the halfway marker in preparation for shooting. This makes the first player have to quickly get back to goal to save the shot.

Play this game until both teams take 15 shots. Then reverse the sides of the field and the side of the goal the players start on.

Notes   Players must shoot by the time they get to the halfway line. As they get tired, they will start shooting early and wildly. Encourage them to get to the halfway line before shooting.

FIGURE 11.13

Setup and execution for Kentucky Derby.

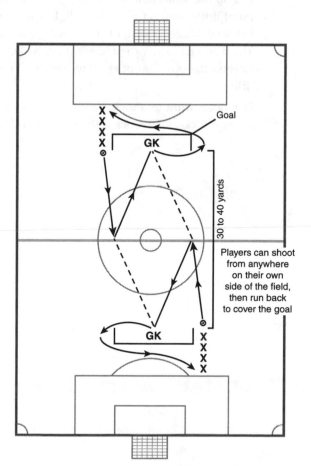

Defensive Games

Marking, tackling, goalkeeping, and providing support on defense are every bit as important as the offensive skills. Here are four games that will help your players sharpen their defensive abilities.

Game One

Name	Slow the Flow
Purpose	To learn how to slow down and properly mark attackers.
Setup	Place players in pairs with a ball and a pair of cones to mark a goal area (see Figure 11.14).
Description	Play this game in rounds of 30 seconds each. One player is the attacker and one is the defender. The defender tries to stop the attacker from scoring. The defender scores a point if the attacker loses the ball, has to turn back from the goal, misses a shot, or runs over the 30-second limit. The defender loses two points if the attacker scores. Reverse the positions after 30 seconds and continue the drill.
Notes	Defenders want to attack the ball and can be beaten by faster attackers. Patience is the key to good marking.

FIGURE 11.14
Setup for Slow
the Flow.

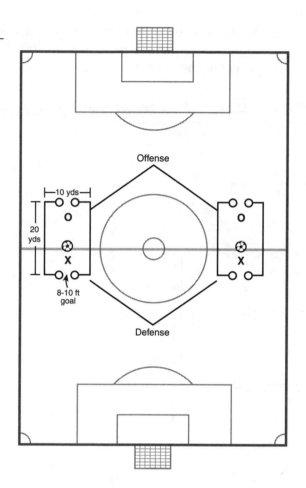

Game Two

Name	Tackle Time
Purpose	To develop timing, aggressiveness, and tackling ability.
Setup	Set up a grid 20 yards × 20 yards. Divide the players into two teams and line them up at opposite ends of the grid (see Figure 11.15).
Description	Give each player a number, using the same numbers for both teams. (For example, if you have six players on each team, you will use the numbers 1–6, with each number corresponding to one player on each team.) When you call out a number, roll a ball down the middle of the grid; the two players run to get it. The players should reach the ball at the same time. If not, make the grid smaller. The object of the drill is to possess the ball by tackling your opponent.

Notes   Most kids like to swipe at the ball and often will miss it. This game emphasizes being aggressive while using proper timing to tackle the ball.

FIGURE 11.15
Setup and execution for Tackle Time.

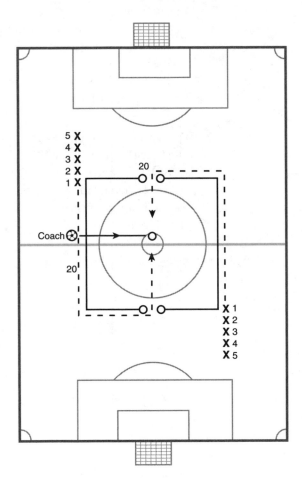

Game Three

Name	Rapid Fire
Purpose	To improve the response time and agility of the goalkeeper.
Setup	Set up two goals and place a goalkeeper in position at each goal (see Figure 11.16). Have your assistant coach supervise one game while you supervise the other. The remaining players are in the center circle; half will be used at one goal, and the other half at the other goal.

Description A player dribbles from the center circle toward the goal he is attacking. Before getting to the penalty area, he takes a right-footed shot. The coach at that goal immediately rolls a ball from the left side, and the player must pop a left-footed shot. The player then turns to the right again and the coach throws a ball in the air that the player heads or volleys into the goal. The goalkeeper has to react quickly to all the shots, going from side to side and coming out on the close balls. Keep this process going until the goalkeeper gets tired; then switch goalkeepers.

Notes The main focus is on goalkeeping skills, not attacking skills. If your players aren't adept enough to challenge the goalkeeper by using the approach described here, alter the approach. For example, each line of players has three balls, and on your whistles (5–10 seconds apart), first Player 1, then Player 2, and finally Player 3 attacks the goal.

FIGURE 11.16

Setup for Rapid Fire.

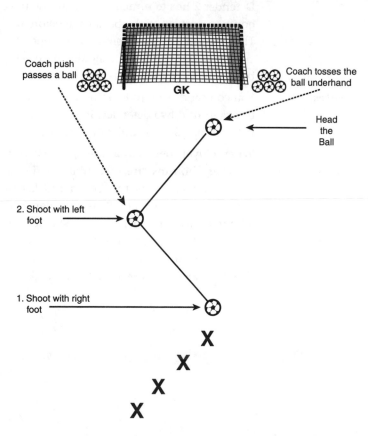

Game Four

Name	Help!
Purpose	To help out on defense and to understand the concepts of timing and spacing.
Setup	Use cones to mark a triangle, with the back cones 10 yards back from the front cone and 20 yards apart (see Figure 11.17). Defender 1 stands by the front cone, and Defender 2 stands on the back line directly behind Defender 1. The attacker, with the ball, stands several yards in front of Defender 1.
Description	The attacker dribbles straight at the first defender and then cuts and runs toward one of the back cones. The object is to get to the back cone first; whoever gets there first scores a point. Defender 1 attempts to tackle the player with the ball but cannot leave the front cone area. Defender 2 has to anticipate which side the attacker is going to and get to the back cone before the attacker does. The attacker has a perceived advantage after he makes his cut to the right or left but should be slower getting to the back cone because he has to control the ball.
Notes	You can set this up in three or four different grids with two attackers and two defenders in each grid. Rotate defenders between positions 1 and 2 and offense and defense.
	When players get good at this, you also can add a second attacker who runs directly behind the first attacker. When the first attacker cuts, the second attacker cuts the opposite way and looks for a pass. The defenders need to decide who takes which attacker. The first defender should take the first attacker, but if the dribbler passes her, the second defender needs to cover the dribbler while the first defender goes to cover the second attacker.

FIGURE 11.17

Setup for Help!

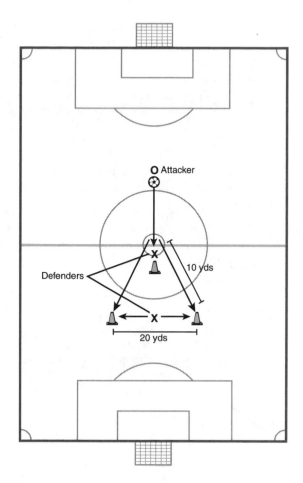

Offensive Games

These two games will help your players hone their abilities to work together as an offensive unit—to move the ball and provide support, to mount an effective attack, and to advance the ball using one of the oldest moves in the book, the give-and-go.

Game One

Name	Side to Side
Purpose	To learn to switch the ball to the opposite side of the field.
Setup	Play on half the field. Form three lines 10–15 yards apart, starting at one end of the field. Begin with the ball with Player B in the middle line (see Figure 11.18).
Description	The player in the middle passes the ball to the player running on his right or left. The player receiving the ball passes

it to the player on the opposite side of the field. This player has options depending on where she is on the field. She can shoot it or cross it to the middle for either of her teammates. All three players should be moving toward the goal and always be prepared to receive the pass.

The object is to move the ball quickly from side to side and attack the goal. When players get good at this drill, add two defenders. Players should rotate positions with each repetition, and the middle player should begin each repetition by passing in the opposite direction from the previous time.

Notes   Don't allow players to dribble the ball in this drill. If players are having difficulty crossing the ball from one side of the field to the other, have them start closer together.

FIGURE 11.18

Setup and execution for Side to Side.

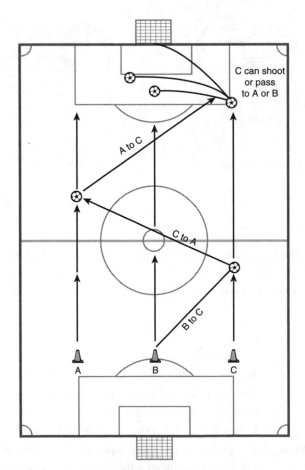

Game Two

Name	Give and Go
Purpose	To help players move to open spaces after they pass the ball.
Setup	Place a series of cones in a line about 4–5 yards apart (see Figure 11.19). Form two lines of players about 6 yards apart, with one ball between them. The players start at one end of the field and move to the other, staying as close to the sideline as they can without going over it.
Description	A pair of players starts on one end, passing the ball to each other between the cones. It's important that the passer passes the ball in front of his teammate and runs to receive the pass back. Each player should have only two touches of the ball: one touch to receive it and one to pass it back. As players get better, they can do it with only one touch of the ball. You call also time them to develop their speed.
Notes	Have players change sides so they are practicing with both feet.

FIGURE 11.19

Setup and execution for Give and Go.

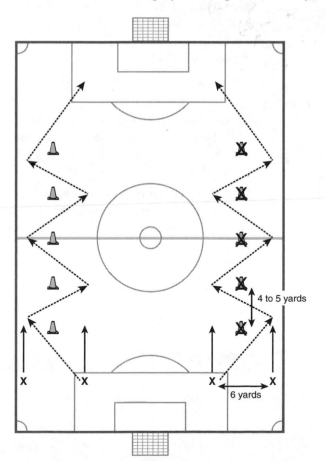

Restart Games

Use these two games to practice effective restarts for corner kicks, penalty kicks, direct and indirect free kicks, and throw-ins.

Game One

Name	Kicks, Kicks, and More Kicks
Purpose	To help players develop the ability to effectively attack on restart situations.
Setup	Place kids in the proper positions for the type of kick they're practicing: corner kicks, penalty kicks, or free kicks (see Figures 11.20, 11.21, and 11.22).
Description	Practice effective attacks with corner kicks, penalty kicks, and free kicks.
	Corner kicks are the most common of all the attacking free kicks. Kickers should try to get the ball about 6–8 yards from the goal line. The other players line up at the top of the penalty area and run in to meet the ball as it comes across the goal.
	For penalty kicks, keeping the kick low and accurate is better than getting it high, even with more power.
	For free kicks, players should try to chip the ball over a wall of defenders to the corner of the goal. This is a difficult skill, however, and only a few of your kids might be able to do this.
Notes	Most kids have difficulty with the timing of corner kicks (getting the receivers moving at the right time to be in the right spot to receive the ball), but it will get better with practice.

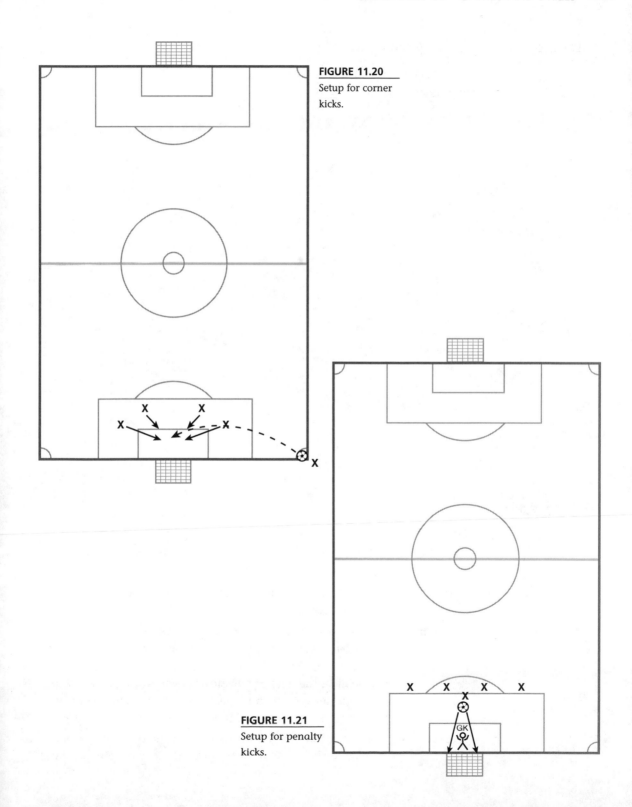

FIGURE 11.20
Setup for corner
kicks.

FIGURE 11.21
Setup for penalty
kicks.

FIGURE 11.22
Setup for free
kicks.

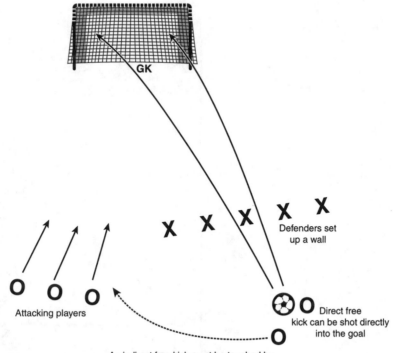

Defenders set
up a wall

Attacking players

Direct free
kick can be shot directly
into the goal

An indirect free kick must be touched by
another player before being shot directly into the goal.

Game Two

Name	Throw and Go
Purpose	To help players understand how to function on a throw-in.
Setup	Place kids in the proper position for a throw-in (see Figure 11.23).
Description	Practice throw-ins at various spots. All throw-ins taken on the defenders' side of the field should be thrown down the sideline toward the opponents' goal, and never in the middle of the field or back toward your own goal. As you get further into the opponents' side of the field, the throw-in can be thrown to the middle of the field.
Notes	The most common fault when throwing the ball in is that players lift their foot off the ground. Have players practice

throw-ins with their feet together. This will help them to not lift their foot off the ground. Also, have players practice throw-ins sitting down; this will develop upper body strength.

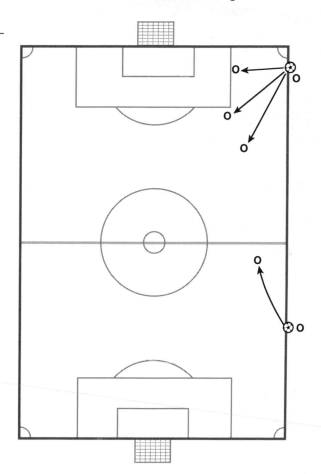

PART III

APPENDIXES

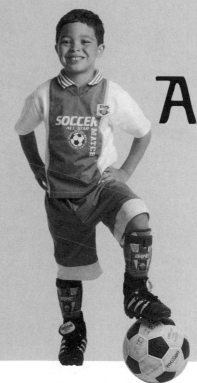

A

SAMPLE LETTER TO PARENTS

Note: This is a sample letter to parents of 6- and 7-year-olds. Your message to parents of older players would likely be a little different. Adjust the letter according to your needs, regardless of the age of your players.

Dear Parent(s):

I'm excited about the new season approaching, and I know you and your child are, too. I want to take a moment to introduce myself and let you know my approach to coaching.

I've been coaching for three years in the park district, beginning when my oldest son entered the league and am certified in first aid/CPR. Over the years, I've developed this coaching philosophy:

- The child is more important than winning. We will do our best to win, but helping each child develop his or her skills, learn more about soccer, and enjoy the experience—while providing for everyone's safety and well-being—take precedence over winning.

- Everyone gets equal playing time. Over the season, your child will play a variety of positions.

- We practice using games and drills that simulate what the players will experience in real games. We do this to practice skills and learn the rules of the game.

- I use positive reinforcement and plenty of encouragement as kids learn the skills. Soccer is a tough sport to master. My focus is to help players learn the fundamental skills and understand the basic rules and strategies of the sport.

What do I expect from the players? I expect them to show up to practice on time, to respect and listen to me, to respect their teammates, to try their hardest, and to have fun. I structure practices so the learning is fun.

What do I expect from parents? I expect them to

- Get their child to practices and games on time or to let me know if they're not coming

- Encourage and support their child and the team during games

- Refrain from booing or making negative remarks to the referees or the other team

- Get involved in a variety of ways with the team (I'll fill you in at the first practice on these opportunities)

- Practice, if at all possible, with their child at home (I'll give you ideas for what to practice)

Please understand that soccer has some inherent risks. I enforce strict rules about behavior at practice, but even so, injuries can occur. These are generally minor, such as scrapes or twisted ankles. I will do everything possible to run an injury-free practice, and I do know how to respond in case of an injury, but I do want you to know the chance of injury always exists in soccer, as in any other sport.

Our first practice is Monday, March 24, 5:30 p.m., at Blair Park. At that practice I will give you a full practice and game schedule. I will also give you a medical information sheet to fill out; this will let me know whether your child has any special medical conditions and who to contact in case of an emergency.

I'm eager for the season to start! See you on March 24.

In the meantime, feel free to contact me at 342-3537 before the first practice, or at any time during the season. Thanks for your attention to this letter, and I look forward to a great season coaching your child!

Sincerely,

[Name, phone number, address]

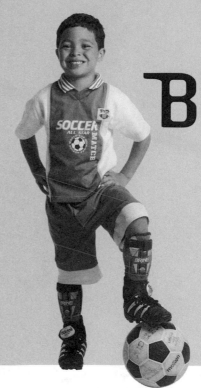

B

MEDICAL EMERGENCY FORM

Child's name _____ D.O.B. _____ Date _____

Address _____ Phone _____

IMPORTANT INFORMATION:

1. Does your child take daily medication? Yes ___ No ___

   If yes, please explain:

   _____

   _____

   _____

2. Does your child have any drug, food, or insect allergies? Yes ___ No ___

   If yes, please explain:

   _____

   _____

   _____

3. Does your child suffer from _____asthma, _____diabetes, or _____epilepsy? Check all that apply.

4. Will your child be bringing any medication to practices or games? Yes ___ No ___

   If yes, please name the medication and explain its purpose:

   _____

   _____

   _____

5. Has your child had a tetanus shot? Yes ___ No ___

6. Is there anything else pertinent regarding your child's health or physical condition? Is yes, please explain:

   _____

   _____

   _____

List two people to contact in case of an emergency:

Parent or guardian's name _____ Home phone _____

Address _____ Work phone _____

Second person's name _____ Home phone _____

Address _____ Work phone _____

Relationship to child _____

Family doctor _____   Phone _____

Family dentist _____   Phone _____

Health plan name _____

Health plan ID# _____

Parent or guardian's signature _____

Date _____

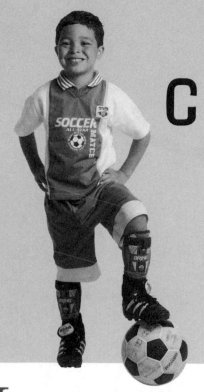

C

INJURY REPORT

Name of child _____

Date _____

Time _____

Description of injury:

_____

_____

_____

_____

_____

_____

First aid administered:

_____

_____

_____

_____

_____

Additional treatment administered:

_____

_____

_____

_____

_____

Referred to:

_____

_____

Signature of person administering first aid:

_____

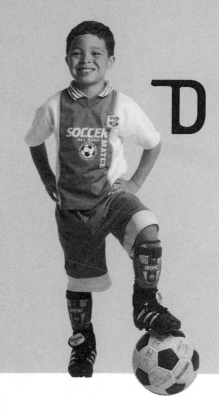

D

SEASON PLAN

Week	Purpose	Tactics/Skills	Rules
1			
2			
3			
4			
5			
6			
7			
8			

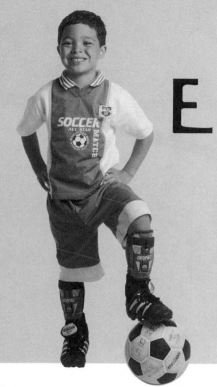

E

PRACTICE PLAN

Date _____ Place _____ Time _____

Equipment _____

Purpose _____

Activity	Description	Time	Comments
1. Warm-up			
2a. STATION 1			
2b. STATION 2			
2c STATION 3			

Activity	Description	Time	Comments
3. Wrap-up			

Notes:

_____

_____

_____

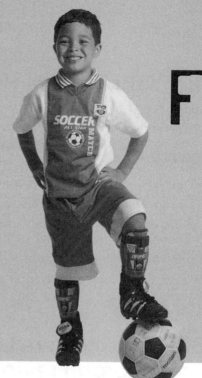

F

SEASON EVALUATiON FORM

Note: Fill this out at season's end. Rate yourself honestly and use this form to note your areas of coaching excellence and areas for improvement for next season.

There are 14 main areas to consider. Respond to each statement made, scoring yourself between 1 and 5, based on this scale:

1 = very poor

2 = poor

3 = average

4 = good

5 = very good

Note that similar statements will appear in more than one area; this is because the issue affects multiple areas.

1. Did Your Players Have Fun?

Statement	Rating: 1–5
The practice and playing environments were positive and enjoyable. I effectively organized practices.	
My players learned the skills they needed to be competitive.	
My players experienced individual successes in practices and games.	
I doled out playing time appropriately.	
I reinforced players' competence and helped them see positive aspects of their performance.	
I didn't overemphasize winning.	
Overall, I would say my players had fun playing soccer this season.	

2. Did Your Players Learn New Skills and Improve on Previously Learned Skills?

Statement	Rating: 1–5
My ability to teach skills enabled my players to learn what they needed to learn.	
I pushed player development of skills at an appropriate rate, neither too fast nor too slow.	
I helped all my players improve and didn't just focus on a certain set of players.	
I adjusted my teaching plan as necessary, according to the skill levels of my players.	
I planned and conducted practices effectively.	
I encouraged and supported my players as they continued their growth.	
Overall, I would say my players learned new skills and improved on any previously learned skills they came in with.	

3. Did You Help Your Players Understand the Game and Its Rules?

Statement	Rating: 1–5
I presented game-like situations for players in practice so they could gain a better understanding of how to respond to similar situations in games.	
I taught my players the appropriate rules and strategies of the game.	
My players showed, through their play, that they understood the basic rules and strategies.	
Overall, I would say I helped my players understand the rules and strategies of soccer.	

4. Did You Communicate Appropriately and Effectively?

Statement	Rating: 1–5
I let parents know my coaching philosophy before the season began.	
I let players and parents know what they could expect from me and what I expected from them.	
I communicated clearly with players, parents, referees, other coaches, and league administrators.	
I kept parents informed and maintained a healthy flow of communication with them throughout the season.	
My players understood my skill instruction.	
My communications with my players were positive and authoritative.	
I was well-prepared for delivering the technical instruction my players needed.	
My players were prepared to respond appropriately in various game situations because I had prepared them for what they would encounter.	
My players paid attention to me when I spoke.	
My body language was in synch with my verbal messages.	
I was a good listener and focused on reading my players' body language and hearing and responding to their comments and questions.	
Overall, I would say I communicated appropriately and effectively with everyone involved.	

5. Did You Provide for Your Players' Safety?

Statement	Rating: 1–5
I was trained in CPR and first aid.	
I warned my players and their parents of the inherent risks of soccer.	
I had a well-stocked first aid kit on hand at practices and games and was prepared to use it.	
I knew of any allergies or other medical conditions of my players and how to respond regarding those conditions.	
I checked the practice and game fields for safety hazards and eliminated those hazards, if possible,before playing on the fields.	
I enforced rules regarding player behavior that enhanced player safety.	
I provided proper supervision throughout each practice.	
I offered proper skill instruction so that players were prepared to play the positions I put them in.	
I took water breaks as appropriate during practice.	
Overall, I would say I adequately provided for my players' safety.	

6. Did You Plan and Conduct Effective Practices?

Statement	Rating: 1–5
Players paid attention to me because I had a purpose to what I was doing.	
There was no down time in practice while I was trying to figure out what to do next.	
Players were active and engaged at multiple stations that I ran simultaneously; they weren't standing around waiting for a turn.	
I used games and drills that were designed to teach a specific skill or tactic that I wanted my players to work on that day.	
My players learned new skills and refined ones they already had.	
My players had fun in practice.	
I had fun, too.	
Overall, I would say I adequately planned and conducted effective practices.	

7. Did Your Players Give Maximum Effort in Practices and Games?

Statement	Rating: 1–5
I didn't yell at players for errors and for their general quality of play.	
I didn't compare one player to another.	
I didn't create long lines in which players had to wait their turn.	
I taught players the skills they needed to know.	
I gave players specific technique goals to work toward.	
I provided specific, positive feedback.	
I encouraged my players, especially when they got down, and praised correct technique and effort.	
I genuinely cared for my players and let them know I cared about them and their achievements.	
I helped players take home the positives of the practice or game.	
I praised hustle, desire, and teamwork shown in practices and games.	
I ran efficient, purposeful practices in which players were active and engaged the whole time.	
I valued each child for his or her own abilities and personality.	
I didn't play favorites with my players.	
I listened to my players.	
Overall, I would say my players gave maximum effort in practices and games.	

8. Did Your Players Leave the Games on the Field?

Statement	Rating: 1–5
I coached my players to keep the game in perspective—to give it their all but to let it go if they lost, and to not get a big head if they won.	
My players were not too high after a victory. They came back prepared to practice and play.	
My players were not too low after a loss. They came back prepared to practice and play.	
I talked appropriately with any of my players who were either too high or too low after a game, helping them to leave the game on the field.	
I talked appropriately with any player who had difficulty mastering his emotions on the field or immediately after a game. I steered the player toward mastering his emotions.	
I helped my players focus on the next game, regardless of the outcome.	
Overall, I would say my players left the games on the field.	

9. Did *You* Leave the Games on the Field?

Statement	Rating: 1–5
I didn't make too much out of a victory. I came back prepared to coach.	
I didn't get too low after a loss. I came back prepared to coach.	
I kept control of my emotions, win or lose.	
Overall, I would say I left the games on the field.	

10. Did You Conduct Yourself Appropriately?

Statement	Rating: 1–5
I communicated in positive ways with opposing coaches and players and with referees.	
I coached within the rules and had my players play within them.	
I maintained control of my emotions in practices and games while providing the coaching and support my players needed.	
I kept the games in perspective and helped my players do the same.	
If I ever lost my cool, I admitted my mistake and apologized for it.	
I was an appropriate role model for my players.Overall, I would say I conducted myself appropriately as a coach.	

11. Did You Communicate Effectively with Parents and Involve Them in Positive Ways?

Statement	Rating: 1–5
I had few or no misunderstandings with parents regarding my coaching philosophy.	
I delegated responsibilities, sharing the workload with many parents and making my program stronger in the process.	
I wasn't as stressed as I might have been, had I not involved parents.	
I appropriately addressed the few misunderstandings or concerns parents had.	
Overall, I would say I communicated effectively with parents and involved them in positive ways.	

12. Did You Coach Appropriately During Games?

Statement	Rating: 1–5

I kept my strategy simple and based it on my players' strengths and abilities.

I helped my players get mentally prepared for a game by focusing them on the fundamentals they needed to execute and on the game plan.

I provided tactical direction and guidance throughout the game.

I was encouraging and supportive.

I gave technique tips and reminders and let the kids play, saving the error correction for the next practice.

I tended to the kids' needs during the game—emotional and psychological as well as mental and physical.

I helped players keep the game in proper perspective.

I used a positive coaching approach.

I effectively rotated players in and out.

My players conducted themselves well during and after the game, including the post-game handshake.

I held a brief post-game meeting, giving the kids some positives to take home, regardless of the outcome of the game.

Overall, I would say I coached appropriately during games.

13. Did You Win with Class and Lose with Dignity?

Statement	Rating: 1–5

I and my players shook hands with the other team, offering them congratulations.

I thanked the referees for volunteering their time.

My team celebrated victories fully and in a way that showed respect for the other team.

My players didn't hang their heads after a loss, no matter how hard the loss was.

I helped the players regroup and take home positives from games we lost.

Overall, I would say we won with class and lost with dignity.

14. Did You Make the Experience Positive, Meaningful, and Fun for Your Players?

Statement	Rating: 1–5
My players still had the same zest and enthusiasm at the end of the season that they did at the beginning.	
My players seemed to want to come back for another season.	
My players learned the skills, tactics, and rules of the game.	
My players learned about themselves, learned what it means to be a member of a team, and grew up a bit.	
Overall, I would say the experience for my players was positive, meaningful, and fun.	

Index

time (playing), 114
touchlines, 36
two-touch passes, 146

under-coaching, signs of, 110

V-Z

warm-ups, 108
warnings, 36
weather guidelines, 70
wingers, 26
winning, emphasis on, 8
winning the ball, 162

zone defense, 164

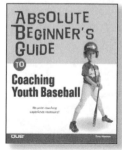
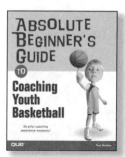
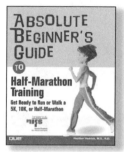
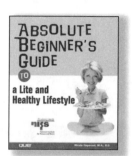
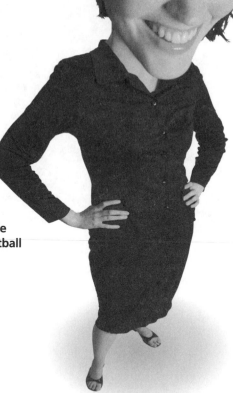

Do Even More
...In No Time

G et ready to cross off those items on your to-do list! *In No Time* helps you tackle the projects that you don't think you have time to finish. With shopping lists and step-by-step instructions, these books get you working toward accomplishing your goals.

Check out these other *In No Time* books, coming soon!

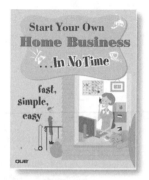

Start Your Own Home Business In No Time
ISBN: **0-7897-3224-6**
$16.95

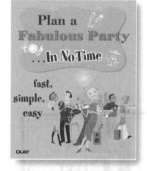

Plan a Fabulous Party In No Time
ISBN: **0-7897-3221-1**
$16.95

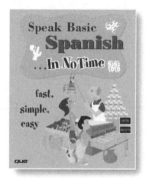

Speak Basic Spanish In No Time
ISBN: **0-7897-3223-8**
$16.95

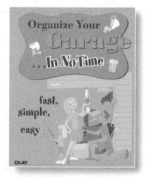

Organize Your Garage In No Time
ISBN: **0-7897-3219-X**
$16.95

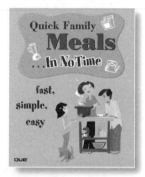

Quick Family Meals In No Time
ISBN: **0-7897-3299-8**
$16.95

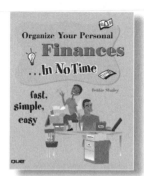

Organize Your Personal Finances In No Time
ISBN: **0-7897-3179-7**
$16.95

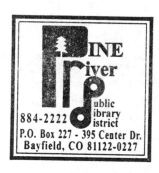